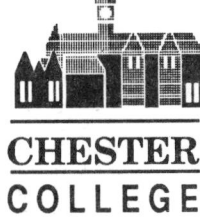

Modern Infectious Disease Epidemiology

Modern Infectious Disease Epidemiology

Johan Giesecke MD, MSc (Applied Mathematics),
MSc (Epidemiology), PhD

Associate Professor of Infectious Diseases,
Karolinska Institute,
Stockholm,
and
Senior Lecturer in Epidemiology,
London School of Hygiene and Tropical Medicine,
London

Edward Arnold
A member of the Hodder Headline Group
LONDON   BOSTON   MELBOURNE   AUCKLAND

© 1994 J. Giesecke

First published in Great Britain 1994

Distributed in the Americas by Little, Brown and Company
34 Beacon Street, Boston, MA 02108

British Library Cataloguing in Publication Data

Available on request

ISBN 0-340-59237-0

Whilst the advice and information given in this book is believed to be true and
accurate at the date of going to press, neither the author nor the publisher can
accept any legal responsibility or liability for any errors or omissions that may be
made. In particular (but without limiting the generality of the preceding dis-
claimer) every effort has been made to check drug dosages; however, it is still
possible that errors have been missed. Furthermore, dosage schedules are
constantly being revised and new side-effects recognized. For these reasons the
reader is strongly urged to consult the drug companies' printed instructions before
administering any of the drugs recommended in this book.

Typeset by GreenGate Publishing Services, Tonbridge, Kent
Printed and bound in Great Britain for Edward Arnold,
a division of Hodder Headline PLC,
338 Euston Road, London NW1 3BH,
by Biddles Limited, Guildford and King's Lynn

Contents

Preface

In many ways, this is the book that I myself would have liked to read some five years ago, when I first became interested in the epidemiology of infectious diseases. At that time, I had been working as an infectious disease physician for several years, and I was becoming particularly curious about the epidemiology of AIDS. How infectious was this disease really? How long did it take from someone becoming infected with HIV until he or she developed AIDS? Why did the epidemic assume so seemingly disparate shapes in different countries and different subpopulations?

When I started to look into the basic literature on epidemiology, I found few books that addressed the issues in the way that I wanted them to be addressed. The authors generally assumed a different perspective, and the examples given in the text had little to do with situations or diseases with which I felt familiar. Conversely, I found that books on the epidemiology of infectious diseases generally dealt more with characteristics of the individual diseases, and that they seldom addressed the methodological and conceptual problems of infectious disease epidemiology *per se.*

Also, quite early in research on AIDS many authors perceived and commented upon the importance of contact patterns for the development of the epidemic. Who meets whom in the population? Few basic textbooks in epidemiology deal with contact patterns in a constructive way, and yet they are crucial to the epidemiology of almost all infectious diseases.

Nevertheless, I slowly worked my way through the literature, often having to re-interpret what I just read to conform with my views and problems. At some time during those years, I had the idea of writing a book better tailored to the epidemiology of infectious diseases. During the academic year 1991–92, I received a scholarship from the Swedish Medical Research Council to learn epidemiology properly at the London School of Hygiene and Tropical Medicine, and during that year the structure of this book began to take shape. The contents – especially as regards collection of illustrative examples from published studies – were completed during my second year at the School, when I somewhat unexpectedly was offered a post as Senior Lecturer in epidemiology for a year. Now, however, I am returning to Sweden, for some time at least, because I believe that any physician who wants to do relevant work in epidemiology has to maintain a strong contact with his or her clinical roots. Without such bonds with the starting place of all epidemiology, one is at peril of loosing one's perspective and sense of direction.

Thanks are due to my friend Professor Gian-Paolo Scalia-Tomba at the Department of Statistics of the University La Sapienza in Rome for having revised and commented on all the statistical parts of the book, making sure that my naïve attitude to statistics did not become too simplified. I am also grateful to Dr. Elizabeth Miller of the Communicable Diseases Surveillance Centre in London for supplying me with the data for the graph on measles incidence in England and Wales in Chapter 10. Furthermore, I want to thank my publishers, *Edward Arnold* and in particular Louise Cook, for the rapid decision to publish and a very supportive attitude. Finally, although for reasons outside our control it has not been possible for him to read the manuscript of this book, I have enjoyed immensely all the stimulating discussions with my boss and friend, Professor Paul Fine, in which he has willingly shared his profound knowledge about the epidemiology of infectious diseases.

When writing this book I have tried to cast my own mind back five years, assuming the knowledge, ideas and misconceptions I had when I started to study epidemiology, and thus trying to write for a reader who is at a similar level now. It is always hard to remember why something was so difficult to understand at first and what the obstacles were. Some of the ideas and examples may not be new to those who already share my fascination for the multifaceted and intellectually challenging field of infectious disease epidemiology, but I hope that other aspects as well as the general structure of this book will prove interesting to them. I also hope that I have been able to transmit some of this fascination to such readers as have not yet seen the light of infectious disease epidemiology.

Johan Giesecke

London and Stockholm, 1994

1 What is special about infectious disease epidemiology?

General ideas about epidemiology are discussed and some reasons are given why you should read a book specifically about the epidemiology of infectious diseases.

This book has been written for people with an interest in infectious diseases who want to learn more about epidemiology. It does not presume any specialist knowledge of infectious disease medicine or microbiology, no more than most practising physicians would have, but the reader should have – or be prepared to start feeling – some sense of fascination about the ever-changing spectrum of human infectious diseases.

I also maintain that the infectious disease perspective is a good place to start learning epidemiology in general, since many of the concepts become clearer and more intuitive when explained with examples from infections. One problem I have found with many, otherwise excellent, introductory texts on epidemiology is that they present the subject more from a public health than from a clinical point of view, and that this tends to make the concepts, terminology, and even examples somewhat unfamiliar to someone with a clinical background.

The book is loosely divided into two parts. The first part begins with a chapter that defines the important terms of infectious disease epidemiology. You may well want to skip it at first, only to return to it when the terms appear later in the text. After this, Chapters 3 to 9 explain concepts and methods that are basic to all branches of epidemiology, such as risk, rate, odds, confounding, bias, sensitivity, specificity, and different types of epidemiological studies, etc. Some basic statistical procedures are also covered. Similar material can be found in other books on epidemiology, the differences being that the perspective here is at times somewhat personal and that the illustrating examples, published and invented, all come from infectious diseases.

The second part applies the tools learnt in the first part to the specific issues of infectious disease epidemiology, such as outbreaks, surveillance, infectiousness, immunity, seroepidemiology, vaccines, etc. Chapter 10 gives the conceptual background for the discussion in the subsequent chapters, and even if you do not like mathematics you should spend some time trying to familiarise yourself with these ideas because they are central to the understanding of many infectious disease phenomena. This part of the book relies heavily on examples from published studies on infectious diseases. The last chapter uses the example of AIDS, which in many ways has the most complex epidemiology of the infectious diseases, to recapitulate most of the topics previously covered in the book. Some of the chapters in this part may also be of interest to persons with previous experience in epidemiology who want to learn more about the specifics of infectious disease epidemiology.

What, then, is epidemiology, and why should one spend time studying it? Basically, epidemiology is about putting people into groups. We are all individuals, and no two patients are ever exactly alike. Even the largest forest consists of trees each of which is unique. However, we all have a number of characteristics that group us with other people: we are either man or woman, we are of a certain age, we live in a certain area, we have certain dietary habits and behaviours, etc., and we share those characteristics with varying numbers of our fellow humans. Epidemiology identifies such groups, ignoring the uniqueness of its members, and tries to discover whether this division of people into groups tells us something more than we could have learnt by just observing each person separately. Since epidemiology is a branch of medicine, our interest is usually to describe, analyse, or understand patterns of disease in the population. The most common situation is when we find one group of people who are ill with some disease, and another group who are not: what is the difference between these groups? Is there some characteristic that seems to differ between them?

On the basic level, epidemiology just starts with a description of the cases of a disease. When do they appear? Where? What ages are they? Is there any other group-defining characteristic that they have in common? Obviously, in such descriptions the individual cases are not of prime interest, but rather the collective pattern of disease that they form. The answers to questions like these may give us clues about a possible aetiology of the disease, or, if the aetiology is already known as in an outbreak of salmonella infection, about possible sources.

In the next step we become more analytical and try to compare systematically the group of disease cases with another group of healthy people. We test the clues offered by the descriptive study by searching for differences in characteristics between the ill and the healthy: did the cases of gastroenteritis eat something that the others did not? Did the children who contracted measles go to a different school from those who did not? Is it more common to find evidence of recent infection with coxsackie virus in children with newly diagnosed diabetes than in healthy children? Will there be more cases of tuberculosis during the next year in a group of HIV-infected people than in a group who test negative for HIV? If our analytical study has been well designed, and if the clues we are investigating are appropriate, we may find strong support for a certain aetiology, a certain pathological mechanism, or a certain source.

The final step is to convert our knowledge about this disease into preventive action. Can hygiene measures be instigated by society? Can we influence people's behaviour to lessen their risk of falling ill? Is there any prophylactic treatment? Could a vaccine be developed? Here again, epidemiology might be called upon to evaluate the effects of preventive measures: did they have the effect on pattern of disease that we had hoped for?

All these steps with the exception of vaccination apply equally to noninfectious and infectious disease epidemiology. There are, however, two features that are quite unique to the infectious diseases:

1. A case may also be a source

2. People may be immune

Concerning the first feature, in most noninfectious disease epidemiology the division between the risk factors for disease and the cases themselves is quite clear. A person's risk of developing coronary heart disease is not influenced by his neighbour's myocardial infarction. Nor does intensive treatment of coronary thrombosis patients in hospital diminish the overall rate of new cases of this disease in the population. For influenza, however, the risk of disease during the coming winter will be greatly affected by the number of influenza patients around, and if many of the people one meets have been vaccinated, the risk of contracting influenza will decrease even if one has not been vaccinated. Treatment of a tuberculosis case will dramatically lessen the risk of disease in members of his family. The fact that a case may be a source also means that the contact pattern in society: who meets whom? how? becomes a very important issue for study.

One could argue that some of the genetic diseases show a similar pattern, where the disease may be passed on from a case to the progeny, but this would be a very particular instance of transmissibility.

The second feature is also unique to infectious diseases. Someone who has had measles will never get it again, even if he finds himself in the middle of an epidemic where everyone susceptible around him contracts measles. For most noninfectious risk factors, such as toxins or radiation, there will be levels when everyone exposed will fall ill. (It could equally be argued that some kind of *resistance* to such risks also exists: why do some people remain healthy after having smoked two packets of cigarettes a day for 50 years? However, very little is known about this type of resistance.)

These two points contain the major differences between the two branches of epidemiology, but there are a few more:

3. A case may be a source without being recognized as a case

By this I mean that asymptomatic, or subclinical, infections play an important role in the epidemiology of many infectious diseases. Ignorance of their existence would make many outbreaks and transmission chains inexplicable.

4. There is sometimes a need for urgency

Most of present noninfectious disease epidemiology concerns itself with environmental and behavioural risk factors for disease. Investigations are often big and lengthy, and their results may enter into public health programmes that often take years to implement. With outbreaks of infectious diseases, the time frame is sometimes more like hours or days before some preventive action has to be decided on. This may give little time for elaborate analyses.

5. Preventive measures (often) have a good scientific basis

Much is known about the bacteria, viruses and other parasites that cause disease, about their transmission, and about how they should be stopped, even if this knowledge may not always have the desired public health impact. Someone who, like myself, has been observing the 20-year debate on the dangers of cholesterol from the sidelines can easily feel content to be in the field of infectious diseases. With some exaggeration, one could say that infectious disease epidemiology is concerned largely with the investigation of preventive factors, whereas noninfectious disease epidemiology is still dealing mainly with risk factors.

Some authors denote what I have termed 'noninfectious' above, 'chronic' disease epidemiology, implying i.a. cancer and cardiovascular disease. This is not very accurate, since several of the infectious diseases are as chronic as many of the noninfectious ones.

One note of caution: I have tried to keep the style of the book simple and as untechnical as possible. The basic common sense ideas of epidemiology should not be obscured by difficult jargon. However, from experience I know that some concepts take longer to grasp than others, and sections may require re-reading once or twice even if the style used in the book makes them seem obvious at first reading.

Another point: the tables and graphs have been placed in the text exactly where they should be looked at. When I read a scientific article I often skip the references to the tables (which are usually on the next page) just to see what will come next in the text proper. I strongly recommend that you do not do likewise when reading this book, but instead give yourself time to study tables and graphs when they appear.

One final thing: a disproportionate number of examples in the book come from studies in which I myself have been involved. This is certainly not because they are better than other people's; it is just that I am very familiar with these studies and for some of the examples I have made use of primary data, which has been easily accessible.

2 Definitions

This chapter deals with a number of the definitions and concepts necessary for understanding the literature on infectious disease epidemiology

Every self-respecting branch of science has to have its own words and concepts. Sometimes it borrows words that have connotations in everyday language and gives them a strict definition with a slightly different meaning. Philosophy, sociology and psychiatry contain a number of such examples, but even within somatic medicine they are not uncommon: A 'positive test result' can mean something quite different to the doctor and to the layman. 'Stress' now denotes a well-defined response from the neuroendocrine system, and not an everyday situation of significant concern.

The purpose of such words is not to deter the novice, but rather to lay a foundation for precise communication. The words of everyday language often have an ambiguity that creates misunderstandings. Some examples:

1. What do we mean by saying that a disease is common? That many have it, or that many will get it?
2. If we say that 'the mortality in disease X is high', do we that mean that X is a common cause of death, or that a large part of those who contract X will die?
3. What does 'infected' mean? That a person is ill, or that he soon will be?
4. If we state that 'the risk of becoming infected with Z is high', do we mean that there is a high probability of meeting someone with Z, or that the risk of transmission is high once we meet someone who demonstrably has Z?

There are a number of definitions that are chiefly or only used in infectious disease epidemiology. The first one concerns the subject itself: sometimes a distinction is made between *communicable* and *infectious* diseases, when the former is a subset of the latter and is taken only to include those diseases that can spread from person to person. In this book we will not make this distinction, but use the terms interchangeably. The John M. Last Dictionary [1] definition of infectious disease is:

> An illness due to a specific infectious agent or its toxic products that arises through transmission of that agent or its products from an infected person, animal, or reservoir to a susceptible host, either directly or indirectly through an intermediate plant or animal host, vector, or the inanimate environment.

Contagious disease is a slightly obsolete term, but if used nowadays it usually means 'highly infectious'.

We will now go on to discuss the most important definitions related to the other specific concepts. Someone who has met with an infectious agent in a way that we know from experience may cause disease has been *exposed*. This definition is somewhat circular, and implies that the concept of exposure relies on present biological knowledge of transmission mechanisms. Someone who passes a patient with Salmonella infection in a corridor has not been exposed to salmonella. A child that has been playing in the same room as another child with *pertussis* has been exposed to whooping cough.

If the infectious agent manages to get a foothold in the exposed person, he becomes *infected*. Sometimes this will lead to changes that are clinically evident or can be assessed by laboratory tests. The most obvious outcome is that he falls ill, i.e. has a *clinical infection*. Frequently, the infected person will not display any symptoms, but can be shown serologically to have reacted to the infectious agent. He has then had a *subclinical* (or asymptomatic) *infection*.

Both types of infection can lead to a *carrier* state for some diseases. A carrier harbours the pathogen - and is able to transmit it - but has no clinical signs of infection. Such a state may be prolonged compared to the acute infection. Examples are hepatitis B and salmonella infections.

The different outcomes of an exposure to an infectious agent are shown in Fig. 2.1.

For a few bacteria a somewhat different carrier state is also possible. The best example are *Staphylococci*, which a person might carry on his skin or in his nose and transmit to others. In this carrier

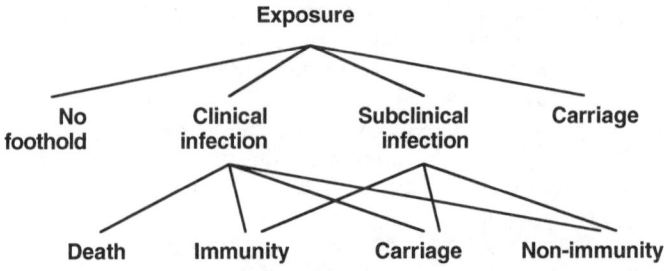

Fig. 2.1 The possible outcomes of an exposure to an infectious agent

state the person is not really infected with the bacteria, but rather locally *colonized*.

The role played by subclinical infections and carrier states in the spread of infectious diseases constitutes an important part of modern infectious disease epidemiology, and is one of the phenomena where this branch of epidemiology most clearly displays its distinctive traits.

Someone who has experienced an infection (clinical or subclinical) with a certain pathogen – or who has been vaccinated against it – so that he shows no clinical signs of infection on renewed exposure to this pathogen, is said to be *immune*. Sometimes it is possible however to show by laboratory methods that an already immune person has reacted to the exposure with an increased antibody titre, and this is called a *natural booster*. Those who are not immune to a disease, and thus potentially infected by an exposure, are called *susceptible*.

An important factor that determines the risk of becoming infected is the *dose*, i.e. the actual number of micro-organisms attacking the person. Whereas a low number of bacteria or virus particles may be fended off directly by the body, a massive dose is almost certain to lead to infection in a susceptible individual.

What is a case?

Much of routine infectious disease epidemiology relies on routine reports of notifiable diseases. Using such figures, cases may be compared over time or between regions/countries. The above list of possible outcomes following an exposure makes it clear that the definition of a *case* is far from simple.

Just consider: to be registered as a case in the classical sense:

The patient

    1. has to experience symptoms from the infection, and
    2. be ill enough to seek medical care or advice.

The physician then has to

    3. suspect the correct diagnosis, and in most cases
    4. send a sample to the laboratory.

The tests in the laboratory

    5. must come out positive, and
    6. the case must be reported.

Finally, the case has to be filed correctly at some central agency.

It is obvious that the number of cases included in the regional/national statistics will underestimate the true number of infections, to varying degrees for different diseases.

The increasing use of laboratory methods for ascertaining sub-clinical diseases complicates the picture even more: If we, for example, start a large screening programme for genital chlamydia infection (which is often asymptomatic), the number of reported chlamydia cases will rise sharply, which might give an impression of a sudden epidemic. Also, for some diseases that are mainly diagnosed through serology, such as hepatitis B and syphilis, there can be ambiguity as to whether the patient represents a new case, or just has markers of an old infection. And, furthermore, even if he can be shown to just have markers of an old infection, he must still have been a case at some point between birth and the present.

Incidence

Incidence is defined as the number of persons who fall ill with a certain disease during a defined time period. If this period is not stated, it is always assumed to be one year: The statement 'the incidence of hepatitis B in Sweden is about 300', thus means that some 300 persons get hepatitis B in Sweden each year. To be able to make comparisons between regions and countries it is customary to divide by the total population of the area. The incidence of meningococcal meningitis in Sweden is about 1 per 100,000 inhabitants and year, whereas in Norway it is several times higher.

Another way of expressing incidence is by giving the percentage of a population that will have the disease during one year. When such percentage figures are given for a disease that leads to immunity after infection, there are two different ways to calculate incidence: either as the percentage infected of the total population, or as the percentage infected of those still susceptible.

In most instances, incidence is calculated from clinical cases, but by following people with serological tests it becomes possible to discover the subclinical cases, and thus to get an incidence figure for the true number of infections.

If incidence is measured over a longer time period, it is often replaced by the term *cumulative incidence*. If we find that 40% of five-year olds have antibodies to varicella virus, we can say that the cumulative incidence during the first five years of life is 40%, but we do not know exactly how the incidence has varied over these years.

Prevalence

The prevalence of a disease is the number of people who have that disease at a specific time. Like the incidence, this figure is often divided by the total population of the region.

A person who falls ill adds one to the incidence of the disease. He will also add one to the prevalence for the duration of his disease, either until he recovers or dies. If the average daily incidence of a disease is called I and the average duration is D days, then the average prevalence, P, will be:

$$P = I \times D$$

or in words: 'prevalence is the product of incidence and duration'.

Most infectious diseases have such a rapid course that 'prevalence' becomes a rather uninteresting measure. Even disregarding the fact that it would be most difficult to count everybody who had, say, campylobacter diarrhoea in a country on any single day, the seasonal variations are so large as to render prevalence figures rather meaningless. The prevalence of influenza A infection in England can be several percents in January for certain years, only to be zero in July.

For chronic or protracted infections, matters become somewhat different. Prevalence figures can be most interesting for hepatitis B carriage, chlamydia infection, or HIV infection. For such diseases, the prevalence gives some indication of the risk of exposure to susceptible individuals. For example, if we assume that a person with acute hepatitis B is infectious during two months, then the prevalence of persons infectious with hepatitis B right now will be the number of carriers plus one sixth of the yearly incidence (assuming an even incidence over the year and also including subclinical infections).

When using serology to determine the percentage of a population that show markers of having had a disease, we often use the term *seroprevalence*. One could argue that this is stretching the term a bit, and that the proportion of a population with markers really is a measure of the cumulative incidence, but that would be too long a term to put *sero-* in front of.

Attack rate

This is defined as the proportion of those exposed to an infectious agent who become (clinically) ill. Obviously, a calculation of an attack rate will depend on how well exposure and disease are measured. If some of the people who were exposed were not counted, the attack rate would be given as too high, and, if instead, some of the cases were missed, the attack rate would appear too low. Also, for most calculations of an attack rate one would want to exclude those exposed who were already immune to the disease.

Primary/secondary cases

For infections that are spread person-to-person, the individual who brings the disease into a population (where the population can be any defined group of people, such as a school class, a group of restaurant visitors, or even a country) is called the *primary* case. The people infected by him/her are called *secondary* cases. If all the secondary cases are infected at about the same time, then the *tertiary* cases will also appear approximately simultaneously, and we can talk about waves, or *generations*, of infection.

Case fatality rate (or ratio)

This is defined as the proportion of people on average who will die of those infected with a certain disease. Usually, one needs some time limit from the start of the illness, and, for example, case fatality rate for measles is often measured as those who die within four to six weeks after the rash appears.

A figure for case fatality rate is largely dependent on how many of the milder cases escape diagnosis. The high figures initially cited for the case fatality rate in haemorrhagic fevers, such as Lassa fever, were probably largely explained by the fact that many of the more benign cases went undetected by the local health authorities.

Mortality

This measure tells what proportion of the entire population die yearly from the disease.

In Western Europe a disease like rabies has high case-fatality rate but low mortality. All the infected die, but the number of deaths is only a few per year. Conversely, influenza A has a low case-fatality rate – most cases survive – but may carry a high mortality. During an influenza season the total number of deaths from all causes per week in a country can be seen to increase markedly. Mortality is thus a product of incidence and case-fatality rate.

Reproductive rate

The potential for a contagious disease to spread from person to person in a population is called *reproductive rate*. It depends not only on the risk of transmission in a contact, but also on how common contacts are: a person with measles who meets no-one will not transmit the infection. In a similar way the rate of acquisition of new sexual partners will influence the spread of sexually transmitted diseases.

The principal determinants of the reproductive rate are:

1. The probability of transmission in a contact between an infected and a susceptible.
2. The frequency of contacts in the population.
3. How long an infected person is infectious.
4. The proportion already immune in the population.

Point 2 above is really the most interesting from an epidemiological point of view, and also the most frequently overlooked. The spread of infectious diseases not only depends on the properties of the pathogen or the host, but in at least equal degree on the contact patterns in the society – who meets whom? how often? what kind of contact do they have?

Vector

A vector is an animal, most often an insect or arthropod, which picks up the pathogen from an infected person and transmits it to a susceptible. The best example is the *Anopheles* mosquito, which is responsible for the spread of malaria.

Transmission routes

Several different classifications for the routes of transmission for different infections exist. This has been done mostly for the purpose of grouping similar diseases together in handbooks on preventive measures, and none of them is entirely satisfactory. Common classifications include: person-to-person spread, airborne, waterborne, foodborne, and vector-borne infections.

An alternative approach could be just to divide the infections into those directly and indirectly transmitted (see Table 2.1).

Table 2.1   *Examples of directly and indirectly transmitted infections*

Direct transmission	Indirect transmission
Mucous membrane to mucous membrane – *sexually transmitted diseases*	Water – *hepatitis A*
	'Proper' air-borne – *chicken pox*
	Food-borne – *salmonella*
Across placenta – *toxoplasmosis*	Vectors – *malaria*
Transplants, incl. blood – *hepatitis B*	Objects – *scarlet fever (toys in a nursery)*
Skin to skin – *herpes type I*	
Sneezes, coughs – *influenza*	

Most of the infections in the indirect group can also spread through direct contact. In fact, the diseases that are placed in the 'indirect' categories are really just the most infectious ones. If you think about it, there are very few infections that could not be transmitted between two people who are so close together as in a sexual intercourse. It is just those pathogens that are so frail that they can only spread through this most intimate of contacts that cause, what we commonly call, sexually transmitted diseases.

The division between sneezes/coughs and 'proper' air-borne has been made to point out that for most air-borne infections one has to be reasonably close to the source, whereas an infection like chicken pox can actually spread from one room to the next through the ventilation system.

Of course, there are also infections that do not spread at all from person to person. Most of these are caused by bacteria living in soil or water, like the causes of tetanus or Legionnaires disease. The epidemiology of such diseases differs very little from the epidemiology of other illnesses caused by inanimate agents in the environment, such as toxins or radiation.

Reservoir versus source

A reservoir is an ecological niche where a pathogen lives and multiplies outside man. Fresh water lakes are reservoirs for *Legionella* . Voles and other small rodents are probably the reservoir for *Borrelia*. Rodent populations of the Himalayans and Rocky Mountains are reservoirs for *Francisella pestis*.

The source is the actual object, animal or person from which the infection is acqured.

Zoonosis

Zoonoses are infections that can spread from vertebrate animals to man. Many salmonella infections are zoonoses, as is rabies. Diseases spread by insects from person to person, but without an animal reservoir are *not* called zoonoses.

There are also a few definitions of time periods that are important:

Incubation period

The incubation period is not a fixed number of days for any disease, but rather an interval, where the middle values are more common than the extremes, and the actual period is often dependent on infectious dose (higher dose usually gives shorter incubation period). The distribution of incubation periods is often skewed left, meaning that there will be more people with short incubation times than with long ones, and references usually give the median (or mean) period, plus minimum and maximum.

The incubation period is from the moment a person is infected until he develops symptoms of disease. During this time he may himself be infectious; in fact, for many of the common childhood diseases the period of greatest infectivity is just towards the end of the incubation period. This fact has important implications for the control of such diseases, since isolation of the cases will often come too late to prevent spread.

Serial interval

For diseases that are spread from person to person, the time between successive generations is called the *serial interval* (or *generation time*). To be exact, this is the time between the appearance of similar symptoms (e.g. rash, cough) in successive generations. Note that if a person is infectious before he develops symptoms, then the serial interval will be shorter than the incubation time.

Infectious period

The length of the time period during which a person can transmit a disease.

Latent period

The period from infection until the infectious period starts.

The relationship between all these time periods is shown in Fig. 2.2 below:

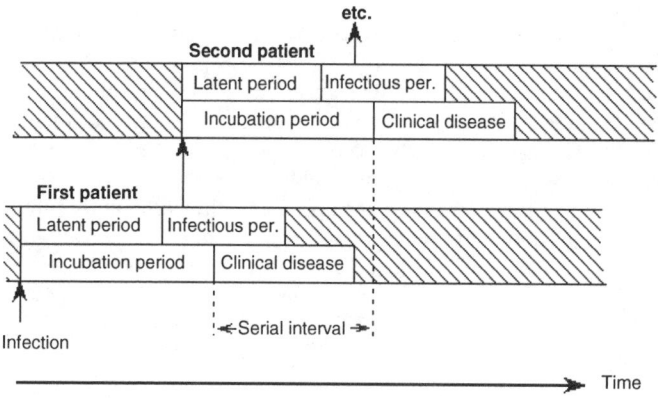

Fig. 2.2 *The relationships of some important time periods. The patient at the bottom is infected first, and transmits the infection to a second patient*

Knowledge about these time periods for different diseases is an important diagnostic aid when dealing with individual patients, but also facilitates tentative diagnoses in outbreak situations, or, if the pathogen causing the outbreak is already known, makes it possible to decide approximately when the exposure must have taken place.

And finally:

Epidemic

This is one of the most difficult definitions of all, and many suggestions have been made. My favourite, and one of the shortest, is the one in Benenson:[2] 'The occurrence of cases of an illness clearly in excess of expectancy'. Some people would probably find this definition too wide, and would like to include something about 'sudden rise in incidence', or 'very large number of cases', whilst others might want to relate it to the public's perception of this health problem. There just is no universally useful definition.

The word 'epidemic' has an ominous ring to it, and many public health officials prefer to replace it with the more neutral term *outbreak* as often as possible.

When an infectious disease lingers at about the same incidence for a long time, we call this an *endemic*. Many childhood infections may be endemic over a couple of years, only to suddenly cause an epidemic every now and then.

There are also diseases that are endemic in some area of the world, but at times spread to other places, causing epidemics. The Ganges area is one such endemic area for cholera, a disease that may become epidemic in other places, like in Latin America in the early 90s. In Chapter 10 we will look at some of the reasons why one disease is endemic, and another epidemic.

For the interested reader, the above-mentioned book by John M. Last[1] is a good epidemiological dictionary, and I have tried to adhere to his definitions in this chapter, adding some personal reflections.

References

1. Last JM *A Dictionary of Epidemiology,* 2nd edition. Oxford: Oxford University Press, 1988.

2. Benenson AS (ed). *Control of Communicable Diseases in Man,* 15th edition. Washington D C: American Public Health Association, 1990.

3 Risk, relative risk, and attack rate

The basic epidemiological concept of comparing risks is introduced, some confusing definitions are discussed, and we meet the attack rate

A not uncommon situation for a practising physician is when several members of a family, a daycare group, or a school class fall ill at almost the same time. Often, the disease is some kind of gastroenteritis, and the patients as well as their doctor wonder if it might have been something they ate. The answer to that question is complicated by the fact that it is not always possible to single out the responsible meal, and even if one could, there are almost always several different food items served during a meal.

An epidemiological analysis of an outbreak

The situation becomes simpler if a group of people who do not ordinarily eat together share a common meal, and some of them become ill afterwards. The following example shows how one could analyse such a situation by calculating risks and relative risks:

Fifteen people had New Year's dinner together. Within 24 hours, five of them fell ill with gastroenteritis. The dinner had consisted of several courses and food items, and the participants had not all eaten the same things. How could the cause of their disease be assessed?

All guests were sent a list of the food that had been served and asked to indicate what they had eaten. As the lists came back, their replies were recorded in a double table, with the ones who had been ill on the left, and the ones who remained well on the right (see Table 3.1):

Table 3.1   *Table filled out from questionnaires given to 15 people during an outbreak of gastroenteritis.*

	Gastroenteritis (5 people)	No Gastroenteritis (10 people)
Quiche	I I	ⅼℍℸ I I I
Cheesecake	I I I I	I
Swiss roll	I I I	I I I I
Chocolate cake	I	I I
Cheese dip	I I I I	ⅼℍℸ I I

The first column tells us that four out of the five people who were ill had eaten cheesecake as well as cheese dip. From the second column we can see that only one of the people who did not become ill had eaten cheesecake, but that most people in this group had also had cheese dip. Just from looking at this table, we get the feeling that the cheesecake may have been the culprit. How can we formalize this feeling?

First we realize that the table is really set up the wrong way. It shows, for example, that if one was ill there was a high chance that one had eaten cheesecake, or that if one was well there was a high chance that one had eaten quiche.

What we really want to know is the opposite question: What was one's chance of being ill if one had eaten cheesecake? Or if one had eaten quiche? We thus rearrange the table (Table 3.2) looking at how many fell ill out of the total who had eaten each item.

Table 3.2   *Number of subjects in Table 3.1 who became ill out of total who ate each item.*

Eaten	Ill	Total
Quiche	2	10
Cheesecake	4	5
Swiss roll	3	7
Chocolate cake	1	3
Cheese dip	4	11

That is, 10 persons had quiche, and two of these became ill, five had cheesecake, and four of these were ill, and so on. From these figures we can calculate the *risk* of becoming ill connected with eating each of these items.

The risk associated with some potentially harmful factor is defined as the proportion who become ill out of all those exposed to it.

Two points about the meaning of the words 'risk' and 'exposed' are necessary here:

1. Note that epidemiology makes a confusing use of the word 'risk'. In everyday language we want a risk to be something that can really cause harm, but in epidemiology it just denotes the statistical chance of being ill if one is exposed to some factor – it says nothing about whether this factor really causes the disease. In the beginning of an analysis we do not know which factors (food items in this case) will prove to be harmful, and initially they are all suspects.

2. The use of the word 'exposure' may be even more frustrating, especially for someone with a background in infectious diseases. Ordinarily, when we say that someone has been 'exposed' to an infectious agent, we mean that he has physically met the bacteria or the virus: someone with influenza has coughed at him, or he has eaten of a dish known to contain *Salmonella*

But epidemiology uses 'exposure' for having met with a risk factor for the disease, which may or may not be the cause. The difference between the two definitions is sometimes subtle, sometimes confusing. Take hepatitis B as an example: known risk factors for acquiring this infection include blood transfusion, intravenous drug use, sexual intercourse, or contact with patients' blood. A person with an acute hepatitis B infection may have been exposed to a number of these risk factors (epidemiological definition), but in only one of these situations was he exposed to the virus (infectious disease definition). The risk factors are 'causal' only if the media involved effectively contain active virus, but they are always 'epidemiological' risk factors, because the media are potential carriers of virus. Another example: someone who has eaten undercooked chicken has been exposed to a risk factor (or has a risk factor) for campylobacter infection, but he may not have been exposed to the bacteria. (Several modern theoretical epidemiologists also advise against the term "risk factor", and propose the much better alternative *determinant*, since this does not imply anything about the cause of the disease. However, this usage is still far from universal, and we will adhere to common terminology here.)

The word 'factor' is also somewhat loosely defined in this text. This is on purpose: it is used to stand for anything that could be associated with risk for disease, a food item, another person, a behaviour and so on.

To get back to the dinner party example: the risk attached to each food item is calculated as

$$\text{Risk} = \frac{\text{Number who ate this food who are ill}}{\text{Total number who ate this food}}$$

i.e. 2/10 for the quiche, 4/5 for the cheesecake, and so on. Risk of illness from eating each one of these things is shown in Fig. 3.1:

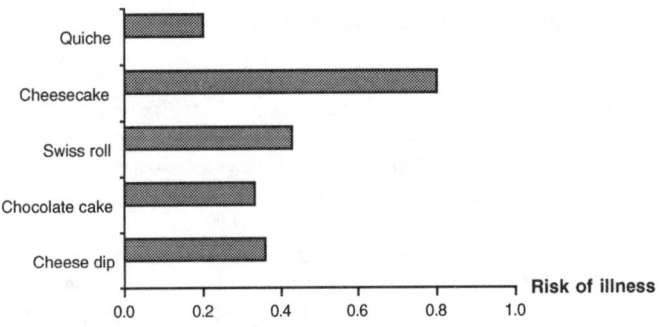

Fig. 3.1   Risk of gastroenteritis after having eaten five different food items.

This gives us a list of possibly infected items, with cheesecake and Swiss roll being most suspect. But let us just stop to think for a while: suppose that the dinner had nothing to do with the five peoples' gastroenteritis, or that the illness was caused by a food item that we forgot to put on the list. The above result may have arisen just by chance.

Now comes the central message of this chapter: we must also look at the risk of being ill in those who did *not* eat the items on the list. We know that almost half of those who had Swiss roll were ill, but what conclusion would we draw if we found the same proportion ill in those who skipped the Swiss roll? The people at the dinner ate many different things, and for most of the items there will be a mixture between those who happened to eat the infected food, and those who did not. If an item was innocent of causing illness, we would expect the same risk of being ill regardless of whether one ate it or not.

This way of thinking is basic to all epidemiology: if an exposure has nothing to do with a disease, then the proportion who are ill after having had this exposure should be the same as in those who had not had the exposure. We will come back to this way of reasoning several times in the book.

We thus proceed to list the outcome according to what people did *not* eat (Table 3.3). Looking at Table 3.1, we can see that three of the ill people did not eat quiche, and that two of the well people also did not eat quiche, and so on:

Table 3.3 *Number of those subjects in Table 3.1 who became ill out of the total who did not eat each item.*

Not eaten	Ill	Total
Quiche	3	5
Cheesecake	1	10
Swiss roll	2	8
Chocolate cake	4	12
Cheese dip	1	4

We can then calculate the risk of being ill if one had *not* eaten each of these items, and put it in a graph together with the risks calculated above (Fig. 3.2):

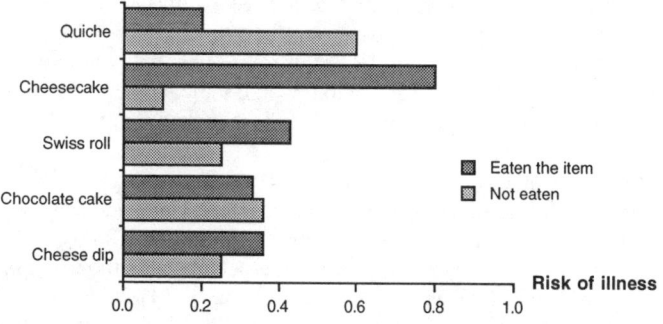

Fig. 3.2 *Risk of gastroenteritis in those who had and those who had not eaten five different food items.*

The figure shows that the risk of being ill is about the same whether or not one ate Swiss roll, chocolate cake, or cheese dip. Eating quiche almost seems to have had a protective effect, whereas cheesecake stands out at the most likely culprit, with a risk of being ill of 0.80 in those who ate it, versus a risk of 0.10 in those who abstained.

A simple way of comparing the risks in those exposed versus those not exposed is to divide them (always putting the risk in exposed on top). This gives the *relative risk* (also called *risk ratio*) RR:

$$RR = \frac{\text{Risk in exposed to a factor}}{\text{Risk in unexposed to this factor}}$$

The relative risks of illness from eating the different food items at the meal are shown in Table 3.4.

Table 3.4   *Relative risk (RRs) of illness associated with each food item during an outbreak of gastroenteritis.*

Food	RR
Quiche	0.33
Cheesecake	8.0
Swiss roll	1.72
Chocolate cake	0.93
Cheese dip	1.44

A relative risk around 1 means that the risk of disease was nearly equal in exposed and unexposed, and that this item is unlikely to have caused disease. A high RR points to this item being associated with the disease, and a RR close to 0 would indicate that the item is in some way protective – the risk of disease is then much higher in those *not* exposed to the item.

From our calculations we find that the RR of causing illness is clearly highest for the cheesecake, and we can conclude with some certainty that this was the item responsible for the gastrointestinal illness.

Two questions remain: why was one person ill without eating cheesecake, and why was one well who had eaten it? There are several plausible answers: maybe the first person was ill from something else, or maybe he ate it and forgot. Epidemiology is rarely an exact science. The other person could simply have eaten so little of the cheesecake that he did not become ill, since risk of infection is often related to the dose of the pathogen.

One may also wonder why the quiche seemed to have a protective effect against illness. One possible explanation is that most guests at the party found it too much to have quiche *and* cheesecake, so that those who had quiche will largely be the same people as those who did not have cheesecake, and who thus escaped infection.

Person-to-person spread

The above is an example of infectious disease that is spread from a common source, and we tried to find a likely cause by comparing relative risks attached to different food items. A quite similar way of reasoning can be applied to diseases that are spread from person to person. We will then want to know the risk of acquiring such a disease from an infected person, i.e. how infectious is it?

For most people this is probably the most important issue regarding communicable diseases, and we all recognize questions like: Can I let my child go to the daycare centre as long as he is infected? What is my risk of getting meningitis now that my neighbour has got it? What is the risk of HIV transmission in a heterosexual intercourse without a condom?

During the years around 1950, Dr Hope Simpson meticulously collected data on all cases of measles, chickenpox, and mumps in a district in western England.[1] One of the things he wanted to study was the risk of transmission from one child in a family to another. To be able to do this he had to register all instances where a child was exposed to a sibling with the disease, and then see how many of these exposures led to a new case. The results during a four-year period are given in Table 3.5.

Table 3.5 Numbers infected out of siblings exposed to three childhood infections.   Source*: Hope Simpson[1]*

	Measles	**Chickenpox**	**Mumps**
Number of children exposed to a sibling with the disease	251	238	218
Number who fell ill	201	172	82

From these figures we can calculate the infectivity of each of these diseases within a family.

The basic measure of infectivity is *attack rate*. The definition is:

The attack rate of a disease is the number of cases, divided by the number of susceptibles exposed

which is really the same as the definition of risk above. The difference is that here we use the infectious disease definition of exposure, by counting only the people who really were exposed to the microbe. The attack rates will be:

$$\text{Measles} \quad \frac{201}{251} = 0.80$$

$$\text{Chicken pox} \quad \frac{172}{238} = 0.72$$

$$\text{Mumps} \quad \frac{82}{218} = 0.38$$

Thus, four out of every five children exposed to measles in the family will themselves contract measles, etc. There is obviously appreciable differences in attack rate for these three diseases.

Likewise, factors influencing attack rate can be studied by looking at number of secondary cases in different groups around a primary case. An obvious such factor is how close one lives to the infected person. In the 1980s there was much concern about the attack rate of monkeypox, since it was known that vaccination against smallpox also protected against monkeypox, but since smallpox had been eradicated this vaccination was no longer necessary. In one study, 147 persons who had caught monkeypox virus from monkeys in Zaire were identified.[2] For each case the investigators counted all the people who had lived in the same residence, and the number of these who became cases. They also tried to calculate the number of more remote contacts that the cases had had, and the number of transmissions to these. The result was:

Secondary Cases		Healthy	
Same residence	More remote	Same residence	More remote
36	11	798	728

so that the attack rate (= risk) in people who shared residence with an infective case was

$$\frac{36}{36 + 798} (\text{total number exposed in denominator}) = 0.043$$

and in the less close contacts $11/739 = 0.015$.

Summary

Whether the number of people who become ill after an exposure is high or low does not only depend on the actual number. It must be compared with the total number who were exposed, and who could have become ill. This is done by calculating the risk. If we want to find out whether an exposure is really related to a disease, we must not only calculate the risk of disease in those exposed, but also in those not exposed. The ratio of these two risks tells us if there is a high probability that the exposure is related to this illness.

When we are looking at a population where we know that all the members have been exposed to a pathogen, the risk of acquiring the disease is called the attack rate.

References

1. Hope Simpson RE. Infectiousness of communicable diseases in the household (measles, chickenpox and mumps). *Lancet* 1952; **2**: 549–54.

2. Fine PEM, Jezek Z, Grab B, Dixon H. The transmission potential of monkeypox virus in human populations. *Int J Epidemiol* 1988; **17**: 643–50.

4 The case-control study: odds, odds ratio. The concept of confounding

The concept of case-control study is introduced and odds ratios are defined. We also meet the 2 × 2 table, and see if an odds ratio for a sample can be extended to apply to a larger group. Finally, we get acquainted with the subject of confounding.

In the example in the previous chapter we had knowledge of the entire population, i.e. we could count precisely how many were exposed and how many were infected. In real life, and especially when studies are based in the community rather than in the clinic, we will often only have information about some of all exposed and ill people. Such a situation requires slightly different methods. Also, in the previous chapter we showed how to give numerical values for different risks, but we did not discuss how exact and reliable these estimates were. For this one needs some statistics.

The first example in this chapter is a published outbreak from Wales.[1] In an outbreak of salmonella infection in a large office block where some 1,400 people worked, 31 cases were identified among employees and six among the staff at the canteen. Only three of these cases actually went to a doctor because of symptoms, the rest were found by culturing of faecal samples, or by interviewing for symptoms.

To compare risk factors with people who had not been ill, 58 randomly chosen employees were given the same questions as the cases. From the dates of first symptoms it was suspected that the infected food had been served on the 23 January. The questions of the investigation were:

1. Did you have lunch in the canteen on 22 January?
2. Did you have lunch in the canteen on 23 January?
3. Did you eat salad on any of these days?
4. Did you eat sandwiches?
5. Did you eat chicken?

The responses to these questions are shown in Table 4.1 below.

Table 4.1   *Results from questionnaires to 37 cases and 58 controls in an outbreak of gastroenteritis in a large office block.*   Source: *Salmon* et al.[1]

Item	Gastroenteritis		No Gastroenteritis	
	Eaten	Not	Eaten	Not
Lunch 22/1	6	31	9	48
Lunch 23/1	18	19	14	43
Salad	12	24	5	52
Sandwiches	16	21	14	44
Chicken	4	33	4	54

In this table, we have included the numbers who did *not* eat each item right from the start, since we know from the previous chapter that we will need them. Also, you can see that there must have been some 'don't remember' here, because there should have been 37 answers for each item in the group with gastroenteritis, and 58 in the group without.

We would now want to calculate risks and RRs just as in the previous chapter, but that is not possible: If you look back at the definition of risk, you see that the denominator should include the *total* number of persons who had eaten the item. In the New Year's dinner example this was easy since we were able to interview everyone who had been to the dinner. In the present example we do not know how many people had lunch in the canteen on each of the days, nor do we know how many ate from the different items on the list. Also, it is unlikely that we identified all the cases; there were probably more employees infected who did not feel ill enough to go to the doctor.

What we have is an unknown proportion of all the employees who were ill, and another unknown proportion of all the ones who remained well. If the symptoms had been more severe, we would probably have collected a larger share of the people who were infected, but we do not know that for certain, and the relative sizes of these proportions are not important for the analysis anyway.

This type of epidemiological analysis is the basic form of a *case-control study*, where risk factors for disease are ascertained by comparing different exposures (in this case type of food eaten) between people who were ill (= the cases) and people who were not (= the controls). In contrast to the study in the previous chapter, we do not have knowledge of all cases, nor of all controls; what we do have are two *samples* of people. Note also that we are doing the analysis 'backwards' in time, starting from a number of cases that we diagnosed, then identifying a number of controls, and after that looking at possible causes of the disease.

Comparisons of risk factors in case-control studies most often make use of the term *odds* . These build on a similar idea as risks, but instead of dividing number of people who were ill by total number exposed, which we do not know, we divide by something we do know, namely the number of people in our study who did not become ill. The odds associated with each item on our list is thus:

$$\text{Odds} = \frac{\text{Number of ill persons exposed to the factor}}{\text{Number of well persons exposed to the factor}}$$

As an example, the odds for the chicken in the table above would be $4/4 = 1$.

Just as with risks, we want to compare the odds for those exposed to the odds for those not exposed. The odds for salmonella infection if one had *not* eaten chicken are $33/54 = 0.61$.

The *odds ratio* (OR) is defined as:

$$\text{OR} = \frac{\text{Odds in those exposed to the factor}}{\text{Odds in those not exposed to the factor}}$$

which for the chicken example would be $1/0.61 = 1.64$.

The definitions of odds and OR are very similar to the ones for risk and RR (so similar, in fact, that they are easily confused, which happens not infrequently in epidemiological literature). Their advantage is that they can be calculated in situations where one does not have knowledge about the entire population. The disadvantage is that they have less intuitive meaning than the words risk and relative risk. Odds do not really *mean* anything, they can just be compared to see which ones are greater or smaller.

We will also at this point introduce the 2×2 (pronounced 'two-by-two') table. It is a cornerstone of all epidemiological research, and often the first thing one draws up when one starts to investigate some data.

The general 2 × 2 table looks like:

	Exposed	**Not exposed**	
Cases	*a*	*b*	*a+b*
Controls	*c*	*d*	*c+d*
	a+c	*b+d*	Total

where

a = number of ill people who were exposed
c = number of well people who were exposed
b = number of ill people who were not exposed
d = number of well people who were not exposed
$a+b$ = total number of cases
$c+d$ = total number of controls
$a+c$ = total number who were exposed
$b+d$ = total number who were not exposed

For an infectious disease with very high infectivity, there would not be any people in squares c and b: All the ill people would be exposed ($= a$), and all the healthy would be unexposed ($= d$).

For the factor 'having had lunch in the canteen on 22nd January', our 2 × 2 table would be:

	Had lunch on the 22nd	**No lunch on the 22nd**	
Ill	6	31	37
Well	9	48	57
	15	79	94

From this table it is easy to calculate the odds and the OR associated with having lunch on the 22nd. The odds of illness in those who had lunch is $6/9 = 0.67$, and the odds of illness in those who did not eat in the canteen that day is $31/48 = 0.65$. The OR for illness for the factor 'lunch in the canteen on the 22nd' is $0.67/0.65 = 1.03$.

Once again: why can we not use the risks from this table ($6/15$ for the exposed and $31/79$ for the unexposed)? No, risks cannot be calculated from these figures, since we know neither the total number who ate or did not eat that day, nor the number of people who were actually infected. We only have our little group of cases and controls, and can only make statements about them. However, if we somehow knew that we happened to have exactly, say, 7% of all cases and 7% of all controls in our study group, then we could have calculated the risks.

Similarly, for the factor 'lunch in canteen on the 23rd', we get:

	Had lunch on the 23rd	No lunch on the 23rd	
Ill	18	19	37
Well	14	43	57
	32	62	94

Here, the odds for illness are $18/14 = 1.29$ and $19/43 = 0.44$ for the exposed and unexposed respectively. That is: among the 94 people who answered this question, there was a considerably greater chance of having had lunch on the 23rd for those who were infected than for those who were well. The OR for illness for 'lunch in canteen on 23rd' is $1.29/0.44 = 2.93$.

In the same way, ORs can be calculated for the three different menu items, and the total list becomes:

Table 4.2   *Odds ratio (OR) for illness associated with each risk factor for the study given in Table 4.1.*

Item	OR
Lunch 22	1.03
Lunch 23	2.93
Salad	5.20
Sandwiches	2.39
Chicken	1.64

An OR of 1 is equivalent to equal odds for disease in those exposed and not exposed to the factor, which is the same as saying that an OR of 1 suggests that this factor is not associated with the disease.

The formula for the odds ratio can be manipulated a little to give an easier way of calculation:

$$OR = \frac{a/c}{b/d} = \frac{ad}{bc}$$

or in words: 'multiply upper left hand number by lower right hand, and divide by the upper right multiplied by the lower left'.

Can we be sure of our ORs?

Our next question is: how far from 1 should the OR be for us to regard the factor as associated with disease? From the list above, we could guess that the lunch on the 22nd probably did not contain any infected food items, but how about the lunch on the 23rd? And should the salad be suspected, with its rather high OR? And as for the chicken?

The answer to this question is statistical. We are looking at samples of cases and controls that may not represent the total population of 1,400 employees perfectly, and it is evident that we could easily just by chance have included too many cases who happened to eat item 'X', or too many controls who did not eat item 'Y'. For each of the numbers in the 2 × 2 table there is thus a statistical uncertainty that affects the exact value of the OR. If the numbers in squares a or d of the 2 × 2 table happen to be higher than they 'should' have been, then our calculated OR will be too high, and if the numbers in b or c are too high, then our OR will be too low. If we somehow could repeat the same study using other groups of cases and controls, the numbers of answers to each of the questions would probably have been a bit different.

The probable range of the true OR can be calculated rather easily from the 2 × 2 table. For each of our five ORs we first calculate something called the *error factor*, which is defined as:

$$\text{Error factor} = e^{2 \times \sqrt{1/a + 1/b + 1/c + 1/d}}$$

(where e is the so-called natural logarithm = 2.71828...).

The formula might seem complicated, but all of the operations can be performed on a simple calculator. As an example, for the exposure 'lunch on the 23rd' the calculation would be:

1. First divide 1 by each of the four numbers in the 2 × 2 table, adding the result to the memory of the calculator each time:

$$\frac{1}{18} + \frac{1}{19} + \frac{1}{14} + \frac{1}{43} = 0.203$$

2. Then take the square root of this number: $\sqrt{0.203} = 0.45$
3. Multiply by 2: $0.45 \times 2 = 0.90$
4. And finally, raise e to this number: $e^{0.90} = 2.46$, which is our error factor.
5. The lower bound of the probable range for the OR for 'lunch on the 23rd' is now defined by dividing our calculated OR in the list above by the error factor:

$$\text{Lower bound} = \frac{2.93}{2.46} = 1.19$$

6. The higher bound is given by multiplying our calculated OR with the error factor:

$$\text{Higher bound} = 2.93 \times 2.46 = 7.21$$

The apparently arbitrary number 2 multiplied with the square root in the formula is chosen to make sure that there is a 95% statistical chance that the true OR lies between the lower and upper bounds, and the interval from 1.19 to 7.21 is called a 95% *confidence interval* for the OR in this example. (To be statistically entirely correct, one should multiply the square root by 1.96 and not by 2 in the formula above to get the exact 95% confidence interval, but this difference is generally slight compared with other measurement and rounding errors.)

You may now wonder why we did not calculate the confidence intervals for the risk ratios in the previous chapter, when we looked at the outbreak? The answer is quite simple: in that example we had the full information for the entire group of people, and the risks and RRs calculated applied exactly to that group and to that meal. The figures were what they were, and could not have been otherwise. In the present example, however, we have taken a *sample* of all possible people in the office block, and it is quite probable that we would have had slightly different values for our ORs if we had taken another group of cases and/or another group of controls. The confidence interval tries to estimate how much chance in choice of cases and controls could influence the range of our calculated OR.

In almost all epidemiological studies, we look at a sample and try to extend the values found to a larger population: a new antibiotic is tested on a group of patients, and the results are extrapolated to apply to all similar patients. The time from infection with HIV to development of AIDS is measured for a group of patients, and extrapolated to apply to all similar HIV-positive persons. Antibodies to measles are measured in a selected sample of children, and extrapolated to apply to all children in the community of that age. In each of these cases we would not need any confidence intervals *if we only wanted to describe exactly the group we have studied*. However, we usually want our results to be more generally useful, and then each group must be seen as just a sample of a larger population, which means that confidence intervals must be calculated.

The list of the 95% confidence intervals for the five ORs calculated above given in Table 4.3 below.

Table 4.3   *Ninety-five per cent confidence intervals for the odds ratios (ORs) for the study given in Table 4.1.*

Item	OR	95% confidence interval
Lunch 22nd	1.03	0.33 – 3.18
Lunch 23rd	2.93	1.21 – 7.09
Salad	5.20	1.65 – 16.4
Sandwiches	2.39	0.99 – 5.80
Chicken	1.64	0.38 – 7.01

Therefore, we can see that for each of our risk factors quite a wide range of values are possible for the true OR. The only two confidence intervals that do not include OR = 1 as a possible value are for 'lunch on the 23rd' and 'salad'.

This result is formulated as: only for these two risk factors is there some statistical evidence that the OR does not differ from 1 just by chance.

(Note: This formula for calculating confidence intervals for an OR is really only valid if all the four values in the 2 × 2 table are equal to 10 or greater. If any of the values are less than 10, the confidence interval calculated will be too narrow. In Chapter 6, we will look at how situations with small values in the 2 × 2 table are handled statistically. Also note that the formula requires the actual numbers of the study. They cannot be substituted by percentages of the groups.)

In this example, as well as in the New Year's dinner example, we have talked about 'exposure to risk factors'. This expression should be interpreted in its broadest sense. There are many types of epidemiological studies where the factors we are looking at could hardly be called exposures. If we want to study how condom usage affects the risk of being infected with HIV, then our dividing factor should be whether or not our subjects used a condom. If we want to compare frequency of infectious mononucleosis in boys and girls, then our dividing variable is gender. If we want to study if chicken pox is a more severe disease in adults than in children, then our dividing variable should be age. Neither condom usage, gender, nor age could really be called exposures.

The most difficult part of a case-control study is often to choose appropriate controls. The cases present themselves, but the controls have somehow to be selected from a suitable population. In this case we just picked 58 people at random from the list of employees, which intuitively seems like a good choice. If, for example, we had chosen employees who never ate at the canteen for controls, our study would have been meaningless. We will return to this question, but the following definition is food for thought: a control should be someone, who, if he had been infected, would have had the same chance of being included as a case in the study as the ones who were actually infected.

Other examples of case-control studies

Apart from outbreak investigations, as exemplified above, case-control studies have relatively rarely been used in infectious disease epidemiology. One reason for this is probably that the method has its greatest use for the rapid screening of a number of potential risk factors for a disease, which is seldom a problem with infectious diseases. There are, however, some noteworthy exceptions. A very nice example comes from an investigation of possible causes for toxic-shock syndrome performed in the USA in 1980.[2]

The disease was named in the late 1970s, when it was found that especially among young adult women there were many cases of a dramatic, rapid disease with high fever, compromised circulation, and confusion which sometimes led to death. At the time of the study, some evidence already pointed to the use of tampons, and especially super-absorbent tampons, as being a risk factor. The investigators telephoned 52 young women who had earlier been diagnosed with toxic-shock syndrome, and asked them if they regularly used tampons during menstruation. Each case was also asked to name a woman friend. The investigators then contacted the 52 friends and asked them the same question. The result was:

	Regular tampon use	No tampon use	
Cases	52	0	52
Friends	44	8	52
	96	8	104

One sees that the odds for disease are $52/44 = 1.18$ in tampon users versus $0/8 = 0$ in non-users, which seems impressive, and it can be calculated that the probability of getting such a difference in odds just by chance is less than 0.02 (see Chapter 6).

Case-control investigations for infectious diseases have, for example, been used to study risk factors for hepatitis C markers,[3] and case-control methods have also been suggested for the study of vaccine efficacy.[4]

Confounding

This is the second central concept of this chapter. The simplest way to think about confounding is like this: imagine that we are looking for risk of disease associated with some factor (e.g. eating cheesecake, not using condoms, attending a daycare centre, etc.). We divide our study population into two groups, one with and one without the risk factor, calculate the odds ratio for disease, and find that the factor seems significantly associated to disease. However, if this factor just happened to be more common in people who had another, *real* risk factor then this division of the population will also get most of the people with the real risk factor into one of the groups. Our finding will then just be a result of the grouping, and the risk factor we were originally looking at may have nothing to do with the disease.

Probably the most commonly cited example of confounding concerns yellow fingers and lung cancer: if one divides the population into those who have yellow fingers and those who have not, one will find that the former group has a much higher risk of getting lung cancer. This association is statistically true, but biologically meaningless. The confounding arises from the fact that having yellow fingers is highly associated to heavy smoking, and our 'yellow fingers group' will thus contain most of the heavy smokers, who have an actual higher risk for lung cancer.

When I was young I was told by my mother not to jump in the piles of fallen leaves that were raked together in the parks in early autumn, because I could contract polio. The observation was statistically true, since the season when there were any piles of leaves to jump in coincided with the time of maximal transmission of polio virus: late summer and early autumn.

Another good example of confounding comes from a case-control study of risk factors for Kaposi's sarcoma in homosexual men published in 1982, before HIV was discovered.[5] At that time it was speculated that the mutagenic effects of the sexual stimulant amyl nitrite ('poppers') might be responsible for the malignancies observed in these men. Comparing lifetime usage of amyl nitrite in 20 cases and 40 controls gave an OR of almost 10 for high versus low frequency of usage, and for several years poppers were discussed as one of the likely causes of AIDS. The confounding comes from the fact that when one collects the men who had frequently used poppers into one group and compares them with the group of men who used poppers less frequently, the former group will also contain most of the men who had had unprotected anal intercourse with many partners, and who therefore ran a high risk of becoming infected by an HIV-positive person.

The problem with confounding is closely linked to the issue of *cause* in epidemiology. One should note that the association between a confounder and a disease may well be perfectly valid statistically, with a high OR and a narrow confidence interval, but still have nothing to do with the real cause of the disease. Another example: suppose that a group of people had a meal where one could choose between fish and meat. The mayonnaise that came with the fish was contaminated with bacteria. When one analysed the ensuing outbreak, one would find a high OR for the mayonnaise, but also for the fish, since almost everyone who had mayonnaise also had fish. The fish would be a confounder, and if everyone who had mayonnaise also had fish, one would not be able to distinguish between these two factors in your analysis. Only if there were some people who ate their fish pure (or who, for some reason, chose to have mayonnaise with their meat) would one be able to see that the fish probably did not cause the outbreak.

If you read other textbooks on epidemiology, you will find that they devote much more space, often entire chapters, to the subject of confounding. Sometimes this tends to make the problem seem more complicated than necessary. Epidemiology is just as much a question of common sense as of rigid definitions and thorny statistics. If you read that coffee drinkers are at higher risk of pancreatic cancer, you should immediately ask yourself: is there some other factor that is more common in coffee drinkers than in non-coffee drinkers? Smoking? Alcohol? The coffee consumption could just be a marker of the real risk behaviour, and thus a confounder.

Another way to think about confounding is to regard it as a question of perspective. Several early studies of risk factors for acquiring hepatitis B infection in Western Europeans used exposure categories such as 'health care work', 'injecting drug use', 'sexual intercourse', which all seem relevant in this connection, but also included 'travel abroad' as a risk factor. Imagine that we made a small case-control study of 18 patients with hepatitis B infection (= cases), and another group of 18 people without clinical or serological signs (= controls), and asked them all if they had travelled abroad. Assume the result was as shown in Fig. 4.1 below.

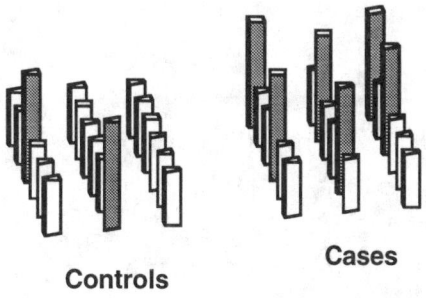

Cases

Controls

Fig. 4.1 *Hypothetical case-control study of 18 hepatitis B cases and 18 controls. A high shaded bar means that the person had been abroad.*

Six out of 18 of the cases had been abroad, and two of the 18 controls. There were thus eight people exposed to the risk factor 'travel abroad', and six of these became cases. Twenty-eight subjects had not travelled abroad, and 12 of these became cases. In this small case-control study the OR associated with the risk factor 'travel abroad' for getting hepatitis B would thus be $(6/2)/(12/16) = 4$.

Let us now change the perspective, and instead ask the question if the subjects had had sexual intercourse with someone who was a hepatitis B carrier (they would probably not know but we will just assume that this information was obtained from somewhere else in a mysterious fashion). The new perspective is shown in Fig. 4.2.

Eight of the cases have this additional risk factor, and two of the controls.

This little example shows that the risk of having had sex with an HBsAg-positive person, which is the real risk, was much higher if one had been abroad, but that the travel in itself is not a risk, just a confounder. The division of the subjects into those who had and had not been abroad puts most of those with the real risk factor in one of the groups (since the prevalence of hepatitis B carriers is higher in many countries outside Europe). Several early studies thus underestimated the role of heterosexual transmission in hepatitis B epidemiology.

If data are collected on possible confounders, it is often possible to adjust for confounding in the analysis of data, as we shall see in later chapters. However, this requires that one realizes what the possible confounders might be, which is again a question of common sense. An analysis could never adjust for confounders that it is not aware of.

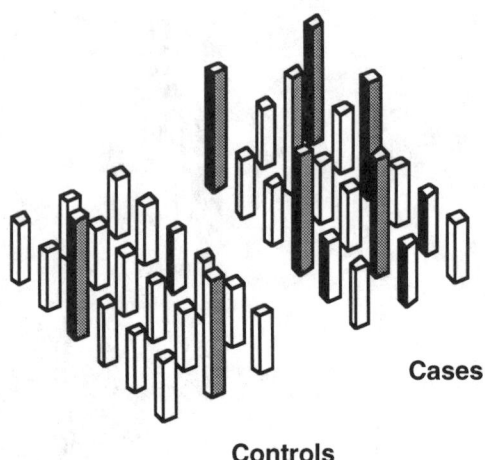

Cases

Controls

Fig. 4.2 *Same study as in Fig. 4.1, this time seen from another angle. Black-sided bars indicate subjects who had had sexual intercourse with an HBsAg-positive partner.*

Summary

If we lack information about the entire population, we can make a case-control study. Risks cannot be calculated, but instead we use odds and odds ratios, which are based on a similar idea.

Since we are only looking at a sample of all possible cases and controls, there is a statistical uncertainty in the exact figures, which is measured by calculating a confidence interval. We say that a factor is significantly associated to disease if the confidence interval around the OR does not include 1. The most difficult part of a case-control study is to choose appropriate controls.

Even if a factor is significantly associated to disease, this may just be a statistical finding, where the division according to exposure also divides the people into high-risk and low-risk groups according to some real risk factor. This is called confounding. The concept of confounding is closely coupled to the concept of cause in epidemiology.

References

1. Salmon RL, Palmer SR, Ribeiro CD, *et al*. How is the source of food poisoning outbreaks established? The example of three consecutive *Salmonella enteritidis* PT4 outbreaks linked to eggs. *J Epidemiol Community Health* 1991; **45**: 266–69.

2. Shands KN, Schmid GP, Dan BB, *et al*. Toxic shock syndrome in menstruating women. *N Engl J Med* 1980; **303**: 1436–42.

3. Alter MJ, Coleman PJ, Alexander WJ, *et al*. Importance of heterosexual activity in the transmission of hepatitis B and non-A, non-B hepatitis. *JAMA* 1989; **262**: 1201–5.

4. Smith PG, Rodrigues LC, Fine PEM. Assessment of the protective efficacy of vaccines against common diseases using case-control and cohort studies. *Int J Epidemiol* 1984; **13**: 87–93.

5. Marmor M, Friedman-Kien A, Laubenstein L, *et al*. Risk factors for Kaposi's sarcoma in homosexual men. *Lancet* 1982; **1**: 1083–86.

5 The cohort study: rates. The concept of bias

The cohort study is introduced and again we look at risks and risk ratios, now showing how confidence intervals are calculated. We also learn what a person-year is, and how it is connected to rates and rate ratios. We then meet the concept of bias, discuss the merits of a controlled, randomized, double-blind clinical trial, and finally make some comparisons between case-control and cohort studies.

The studies we have been looking at in the two previous chapters have all analysed an epidemiological pattern *after* the event has occurred. Sometimes one may be able to plan an epidemiological study a little better in advance. Such studies, where a defined group of people are followed over time, are probably more familiar to most clinicians than case-control studies.

In a study of HIV infection and tuberculosis in New York,[1] 513 intravenous drug users were initially tested for HIV antibody. Two hundred and fifteen were HIV positive and 298 HIV negative. They were then followed for any signs of active tuberculosis during an average of two years. The results of the study were:

	HIV seropositive initially	HIV seronegative initially	
Developed TB	8	0	8
No TB	207	298	505
	215	298	513

The risk of developing tuberculosis in this group was thus 8/215 = 0.037 for those who were seropositive at entry, and 0/298 = 0 for those who were seronegative.

This type of study, where one first defines and measures the risk factor one wants to evaluate (in this case HIV status) in a defined group, and then follows this group over time to see who develops disease (in this case TB) is called a *cohort study*.

Another example: there has been much discussion about whether sexually transmitted diseases, and especially genital ulcerative disease, increase the risk of HIV transmission. In a study from Nairobi,[2] Cameron, *et al.* followed 291 men who presented at an STD clinic. They all reported to have had sexual intercourse with women from a group of prostitutes where HIV infection was known to be common. About half of the men presented with an ulcerative disease, the rest with urethritis. After the first visit, the men were tested repeatedly for three months, to see if they had also seroconverted in an HIV antibody test (which may take several weeks to become positive after the actual transmission). The result was:

	Presented with genital ulcers	Presented with another condition	
Seroconverted	21	3	24
Remained HIV-negative	128	141	269
	149	144	293

The RR of seroconversion for the factor 'ulcerative disease' was thus:

$$\frac{21/149}{3/144} = 6.8$$

The authors concluded that the men infected with ulcerative disease were infected with HIV in the same intercourse, and that women who had an ulcerative disease were also more likely to transmit the HIV virus.

In a cohort study, we can always use risks and RRs for our comparisons, since we have started by defining the total group of people that we want to study.

In a similar fashion as with the ORs of the previous chapter, we need some way of deciding the precision of our calculated RRs. We need to know how much the 'true' RR could differ from the one we have found, and specifically if it is possible that the RR could be 1 (which would mean that we cannot deduce that the factor we are analysing is associated with disease).

The way of calculating a confidence interval for an RR is almost the same as for an OR. We first calculate the error factor:

$$\text{Error factor} = e^{2\times\sqrt{1/a+1/b}}$$

and then divide and multiply the RR with this value to get the lower and upper bounds, respectively. (One may wonder why the last two terms under the root sign are 'missing' here, compared with the error factor for the OR. Simply put, this is because in a cohort study, the exact number of people in both groups is fixed from the start, and therefore there is no chance variation in these numbers, as there was for c and d in the case-control study.)

For the RR of the Nairobi study, a very approximate calculation would be:

$$\text{Error factor} = e^{2\times\sqrt{1/a+1/b}} = e^{2\times\sqrt{1/21+1/3}} = e^{2\times0.62} = 3.46$$

and the lower and upper bound for our confidence interval 6.8/3.46 = 1.97, and 6.8 × 3.46 = 23.5, respectively. The confidence interval thus seems to be well above RR = 1, but since the formula above requires that both a and b are at least 10, this approximate interval cannot be trusted entirely.

A cohort study does not have to be *prospective*, i.e. a study where the subjects are entered at that time and subsequently followed into the future. If there is a way of collecting a cohort that was defined at some time in the past, it is possible to save a lot of time by looking at its members now. This could be called a *retrospective* cohort study.

There has been some debate whether acute infectious myocarditis predisposes for chronic cardiomyopathy with heart failure later in life. In a study undertaken in 1986,[3] 44 of the 45 patients that had been hospitalized at one hospital in Stockholm for acute myocarditis in 1968 and 1969 were contacted. They had then been part of a study to ascertain the microbiological aetiology of their condition, and had been diagnosed and investigated rigorously. Just by sending them a questionnaire it was possible to show that their risk of having any heart disease was not different from that of the average population. In this way, a 17-year follow-up was accomplished in a few months.

This study used the average population as the nonexposed group, which is quite common in cohort studies. In doing so, one implicitly assumes that the proportion exposed to the risk factor in the average population is low. Ideally, the control group should only consist of people who had never been exposed to the risk factor (i.e. who had never had myocarditis in this case), but this condition is difficult to meet when one uses published national health statistics for the comparison. If, however, the disease is rare, the influence from the few exposed individuals on the overall frequency of the disease in the overall population will be very diluted.

Different follow-up times

One problem in the analysis of cohort studies is that all subjects are rarely observed for the same time period. They may enter the study at different times and they may be lost to follow-up at different times. In a large study over a long time, it is inevitable that the investigators loose contact with some of the individuals.

The way to deal with this is not to use the number of persons in the exposed and unexposed groups for the calculation of risks, but the sum of times each person has been followed up. Therefore, for each individual in the study one measures the time from entry either until he becomes ill, or until he is lost to follow-up, or until the study is terminated. This time becomes the observation period for each person, and these times are added for all people in each group. Most often, number of months or years are added, and the number of people who become ill is divided by number of person-months or person-years experienced by all subjects in the group. Fig. 5.1 below illustrates this principle.

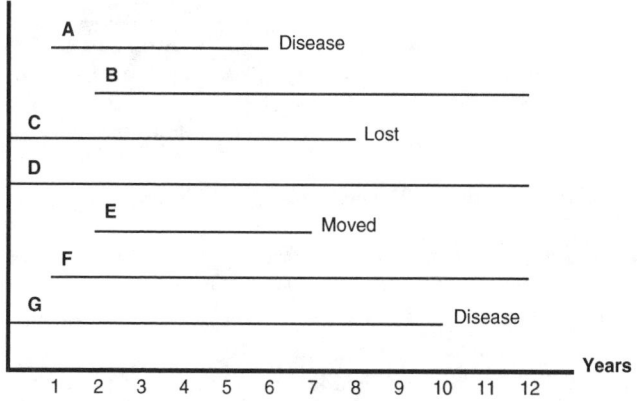

Fig. 5.1 Schematic representation of a cohort study. Each line, A to G, represents the monitoring period for a patient.

Seven people who are at risk for some disease are followed in a cohort study that lasts 12 years. Subject A enters the study after one year, and becomes ill after six years. He contributes five person-years. Subject B enters after two years, and is still well at the end of the study, thus adding 10 years. Subject C is followed from the start, but the investigators loose contact with him after eight years, and so on. The total number of person-years in this study would be:

$$5 + 10 + 8 + 12 + 5 + 11 + 10 = 61.$$

Risks and rates

One of the most abused words in epidemiology is *rate*. This word should mean something that has to do with changes over time, i.e. how quickly something is happening. It is, however, very often taken to mean just 'proportion', or 'percentage'. This practice is confusing to the novice entering the field of epidemiology, and should be discouraged. (Though for some concepts, such a change in terminology will probably be a long time coming: a good example is the term 'attack rate' which we met in Chapters 2 and 3. This is not a rate at all, but rather a proportion or a percentage.)

Here, we need *rate* in its proper sense to describe the situation in Fig. 5.1 because if you look back to the definition of risk in Chapter 3, it is: 'the proportion who become ill out of all those exposed to a factor'. This definition is clear for an outbreak, when everyone who became ill did so within 24 hours, but what happens if we follow exposures and diseases over much longer periods? The long-term risk of dying after exposure to any risk factor is always 100%, because as the author says, 'in the long run we are all dead'. In most situations, the risk of becoming infected with a pathogen that exists around us, like herpes, TB, or campylobacter, is evidently greater the longer the time interval one considers. In short: the figure for a risk depends on the time period.

This problem does not adhere to the concept of a rate. It is defined thus:

> The **rate** is the number who fall ill, divided by the total time under study added by all the subjects in the cohort.

In Fig. 5.1 above, there are two persons who acquire the disease during the 61 person-years of the study. The rate is calculated as the number who become ill, divided by total number of person-years, or in this case $2/61 = 0.033$ per person-year. In using a rate, we assume that all person-years are comparable, so that there will be the same number of cases if we follow 100 subjects during one year as if we follow 10 persons for 10 years (the predicted number of cases in this example being 3.3 for both studies).

If the people in the figure were patients who were HBsAg-positive, and the disease was cirrhosis, we could compare them to another group of people who were HBsAg-negative, and calculate the rate of development of disease in that group. Just like for RR and OR, we could then divide them to yield a *rate ratio*, which would show by how much HBsAg positivity increased the rate of acquiring cirrhosis.

The confidence interval for a rate ratio is calculated just as for an RR, i.e. by first getting the error factor

$$EF = e^{2 \times \sqrt{1/a + 1/b}}$$

where a is the number of people who fall ill in the first group, and b the number in the second (both should be greater than 10 for the formula to apply properly). The rate ratio is then divided by the EF to get the lower bound, and multiplied with it to get the upper.

Bias

Bias is probably a much more familiar concept to most clinicians than confounding. It has to do with the representativity of our subjects and our data: are the patients in the study really a good sample of all the patients we want to make inferences about? Is the same attention given to the subjects in the case group and the control group? Do the subjects in both groups respond to our questions with equal honesty?

The ability to discover possible biases requires a combination of common sense and clinical experience. Some examples:

1. It would obviously be misleading to use the patients with salmonella in an infectious disease ward for a study of the clinical symptoms and complication risks of a salmonella infection. These patients would be much more seriously ill than the average salmonella infection case (since they were referred to a hospital).
2. The proportion of people infected with HIV in a country can hardly be estimated by the percentage of HIV-positive blood donors. Since people who can be suspected to be at high risk of HIV infection are actively discouraged from donating blood, this figure must surely be an underestimate.
3. People given a new vaccine will be closely scrutinized for adverse reactions. If we do not follow a comparison group that

should ideally be injected with distilled water or some other inert substance just as closely, we are liable to overestimate the risk of mild adverse reactions in the group given the new treatment (since many mild reactions, such as headache or general *malaise* may have nothing to do with the vaccine, and should be just as common in the control group).

4. In a case-control study of an outbreak, the cases are probably more likely to remember just what they ate, since they will already have suspected the meal, and may have thought through, or talked through, the different possible dishes responsible.

Examples 1 and 2 represent *selection biases*, example 3 represents an *observer bias*, and 4 a *response bias*. When you design a study, or read one that has been published, you should use your experience and carefully consider the different biases possible.

Clinical trials

A clinical trial is really a special example of a cohort study. The major conceptual difference between an epidemiological study and a clinical trial is that in epidemiology we generally cannot control the risk factors or exposures of the subjects; we have to be satisfied with the way nature or chance has set up the 'experiment' for us. In clinical trials, on the other hand, we can choose the subjects at will, and also assign different exposures (most often types of treatment) to different groups.

The golden standard of all such research is the *placebo-controlled, randomized, double-blind* clinical trial. Reflecting on the merits of this research strategy gives good practice in thinking about confounding and bias. Let us look at each of these three terms:

Placebo-controlled

When we subject a group of patients to a new treatment, we can usually observe changes. The patients may be feeling better, they may have lower values for their liver enzymes, or they may be able to leave the hospital earlier. The problem is that we often cannot be sure that these improvements are not caused by chance, or by something else that changed since we started the treatment. If the improvement is really due to some other concurrent change in treatment, we would have a good example of confounding: The difference in outcome that we ascribe to our new treatment is really explained by some associated event.

The way to solve this problem is to have a *control* group of patients with the same disease, who receive exactly the same treatment as the study patients, except for the factor we want to study. Ideally they should be given some inactive treatment (which is called *placebo*), or the previously best available treatment. The situation is rather like the comparison of risk of gastroenteritis from eating cheese cake in Chapter 3, where the group who did not eat cheese-cake supplied a measure of risk of disease in the control group. In any clinical trial, the changes in the group on active treatment should be compared to the control group to see if the differences indicate a real effect.

Several studies have shown a so called 'placebo effect' of some 30% in clinical trials, which means that around 30% of patients will experience some effect even from totally inactive substances. Probable explanations for this are simply people's expectations, or the increased attention they get from their doctor when they are subjects of some kind of trial.

Randomized

When we have a group of patients, and want to assign them to two (or more) different treatments, a number of biases are possible. If we let the patient choose treatment, it is conceivable that certain types of patients will choose certain options, which could mean that the groups do not become similar in other important variables. If the physician makes the choice, he might allocate patients to the different groups according to his preconceptions of the new treatment: if he believes strongly in the new therapy, there may be a tendency to allocate the really ill patients to the treatment group, but if he is uncertain about its merits, it may be the other way around.

Randomization assures that there is no bias as to which patient gets which treatment. If the groups are large enough, it also tends, just by chance, to make the two groups similar in all variables that may cause confounding, such as age, sex, etc. For small groups this may not be the case, and one should always in the analysis check that the groups are comparable as regards possible confounders (same average age, equal proportion of men/women, etc.).

Double-blind

The word 'blinding' implies being ignorant of whether or not the patient is taking the active drug. 'Single-blind' means that the patient does not know, but that the physician does. In a 'double-blind' trial, neither of them knows. There is even something called 'triple-blind' trials, where the statistician evaluating the outcome of the study is also kept ignorant about the meaning of the group assignments until after the analysis is completed.

Blinding may be important, since even if there is a good control group and treatment has been randomized, there is still the chance that the patient's or the physician's preconceptions about the new therapy will influence the results. This is especially a problem when outcome variables are more or less subjective, as with, for example, insomnia or headache, but even if the variables measured are 'hard figures', physician knowledge of allocation group may still influence frequency of blood tests or interpretation of borderline values.

By assuring that both physician and patient are blind to which group the patients belong, such biases can be eliminated. Double blinding is, of course, only possible when there is an alternative therapy that cannot be distinguished from the one under trial, i.e. almost exclusively in tests of drugs. A study of surgery versus antibiotic therapy in the treatment of brain abscess can hardly be blinded. Even in placebo-controlled tests of drugs, it may often be possible for the physician to guess if the patient is on active treatment or not from the results of blood chemistry. Thus, trials of zidovudine for HIV infection have been criticized on the grounds that this drug increases the volume of the red blood cells, which can easily be seen from an ordinary haemoglobin count and haemocrit. This would in fact make the study only single-blind.

Pro's and con's of case-control and cohort studies

This and the previous chapters have introduced the concepts of case-control and cohort studies. It may not be entirely clear why sometimes the one is chosen for an epidemiological study and sometimes the other.

One important conceptual difference between the two types of study has to do with time: in a cohort study we start with a number of subjects who are free from disease, and follow them over time to see who becomes a case and who does not. In a case-control study, the events have already happened before the study started, and we collect the cases and try to find appropriate, disease-free controls.

This means that in many instances the choice of method is actually governed by the available data. Cohort studies usually require carefully planned, often lengthy investigations, whilst a case-control study can quite often be performed quickly from a number of cases already collected.

Another important deciding factor concerns the incidence of the disease one wishes to study. For diseases with a very low incidence, cohort studies may not be practical, or even feasible. Suppose we had a suspicion that the use of dental floss is a strong risk factor for developing infectious endocarditis: the repeated small traumas to the gums from pulling these plastic bands back and forth between the teeth could serve as portals of entry into the blood stream for the alpha streptococci of the mouth. Endocarditis is a very rare disease, and it seems quite clear that most people who use dental floss do not develop it. If we wanted to study this question in a cohort fashion, we would probably need to collect one huge group of dental floss users and one of non-users, and then follow them for a long time to see if any cases of endocarditis appeared. It is doubtful if such a study would be feasible. In the case-control mode, we would instead approach a number of people already diagnosed with endocarditis and ask them if they were dental floss users. We would then calculate the proportion of 'yes' answers in this group and com-pare the result to the proportion of users in a similar group of people who had not had endocarditis, and so attain an odds ratio for usage in the group of cases. The latter approach would obviously be very much faster and cheaper.

If on the other hand the incidence of the disease is high, it might be just as easy to collect a cohort and follow them as to get into the delicate business of finding adequate controls. This is especially true as problems with bias and confounding are often worse in a case-control than in a cohort study. If we wanted to study the efficacy of an influenza vaccine during an epidemic season, the simplest way would probably be to randomly vaccinate half of a defined group of people and follow the entire group for a couple of months. A case-control study in this situation would mean comparing vaccination status in cases and non-cases of influenza, and it could be difficult to make certain for example that there were no confounding factors as to who had been vaccinated or not.

Another principal conceptual difference concerns the measures of strength of association in the two types of studies: the ORs and the RRs. As was pointed out in Chapter 4, an odds ratio does not have any directly interpretable meaning, it just tells us how strongly an exposure and an outcome seem to be related. In the example with dental floss above, a case-control study might reveal a very strong and statistically significant relationship between floss usage and endocarditis. But this OR would not tell us what we really want to know: what is my risk of developing endocarditis if I use dental floss regularly for, say, thirty years? To answer this question, we need a study that could measure the risks, and we are left with the option of an impossible cohort study.

However, theoretical developments in epidemiology during the last decades have shown that in some instances the OR attained from a well-performed case-control study could serve as a good approximation to the usually more relevant RR. This is especially true if the disease is rare both in those who have the risk factor and those who have not, which can be shown by looking at the general 2×2 table again:

	Exposed	Not exposed	
Ill	a	b	$a+b$
Healthy	c	d	$c+d$
	$a+c$	$b+d$	

If this had been the result of a regular cohort study, we would have said that the risk of disease in the exposed was $a/(a + c)$ and in the not exposed $b/(b + d)$. The relative risk of becoming ill for someone who was exposed would be

$$RR = \frac{\dfrac{a}{a+c}}{\dfrac{b}{b+d}} = \frac{a(b+d)}{b(a+c)}$$

However, if this was a rare disease, this means that in the total population the number of unexposed ill people *(b)* would be very small compared with the large number of unexposed healthy people *(d)*. The sum *(b + d)* would thus almost be the same as *d* only. Likewise, the number of exposed people who became ill *(a)* would be very small compared to all the people who were exposed but remained healthy *(c)*, and thus *(a + c)* $\approx$ *c*.

The relative risk of disease would accordingly be

$$\frac{a(b+d)}{b(a+c)} \approx \frac{ad}{bc}$$

which is the definition of the odds ratio. Thus, for rare diseases, the OR often provides a good approximation of the RR.

It can, in fact, be shown that depending on how the controls are chosen, we can get an OR that is an estimate either of the classical odds ratio, or of the relative risk, or of the rate ratio even for diseases that are not rare.[4] I will not go into the details of those theoretical discussions here, but just point out that the times at which the controls are chosen are important.

In a 'classical' case-control study, one collects a set of cases and then looks around for disease-free controls. These should hopefully be selected in a way that avoids biases, and data on possible confounders should be recorded. Another way of choosing could be to identify a control for each case just at the time when the case falls ill. This means that a person who was originally chosen as a control could well become a case later, but that does not disqualify him from remaining as a control in the study. It can be shown that an OR calculated from such a study becomes a good approximation of the rate ratio of disease between exposed and nonexposed.

One note of caution, however, concerning the use of case-control studies to estimate relative risks and rates. Even if the methods suggested seem attractive and have good theoretical foundations, they still always assume completely unbiased choice of controls. Probably the most important condition is that the selection of cases and controls should not be based on exposure status, or stated even more formally: the exposure distribution in the controls should be an unbiased estimate of the exposure distribution in the general population. When reading the results of any case-control study, one should always ask: how were the cases selected? How were the controls selected? Could there be any systematic difference between the two selections, so that the groups are not really representative of the same population?

The final deciding factor in choosing type of study is not seldom cost. There is a well-known joke among epidemiologists that says: 'No researcher will ever be able to undertake a cohort study, since when one is old and recognized enough to get the large funds necessary, one will be too close to retirement to be able to follow the project to completion, and when one is sufficiently young to have time to see the project through, one will be too unproven to get the kind of research money that is needed.'

Summary

In cohort studies we follow defined groups of people over time to see how many develop disease. By dividing this figure with the original number of subjects we calculate the actual risk of disease in each group. In real life, the subjects of a cohort study often enter at different times, and it becomes practical to use the total time in the study, i.e. person-years or person-months, to calculate what proportion fall ill per person-time unit, which is then called the rate.

Cohort studies often take a long time, and it is important that all the participants are followed up for the entire study, or at least that the causes of loss to follow-up are known for each subject. If we selectively loose contact more with one group of subjects than the other, for example, if the people we denote as 'losses to follow-up' have in reality died from the disease we are studying, then our estimate of risk or rate will be biased.

Bias may be introduced by the selection of subjects or by the way data is collected. Avoidance of bias requires careful consideration when a study is planned. Once it has been introduced, it may be impossible to adjust for it in the analysis of data.

A controlled, randomized, double-blind trial tries to get rid of confounders (known and unknown) and of biases by letting chance decide who gets into which group, and by precluding patient and observer bias. If confounding variables are to be equally distributed between the groups, these cannot be too small, since chance may easily play tricks with small numbers.

The choice between performing a cohort or a case-control study is often governed by considerations of time and money. Generally, cohort studies have less problem with bias, but are more time-consuming and expensive.

References

1. Selwyn PA, Hartel D, Lewis VA, *et al*. Prospective study of tuberculosis among intravenous drug users with human immunodeficiency virus infection. *N Engl J Med* 1989; **320**: 545–50.

2. Cameron DW, Simonsen JN, Lourdes JD, *et al*. Female to male transmission of human immunodeficiency virus type 1: risk factors for seroconversion in men. *Lancet* 1989; **2**: 403–7.

3. Giesecke J. The long-term prognosis in acute myocarditis. *Eur Heart J* 1987; **8**: 251–53.

4. Rodrigues L, Kirkwood B. Case-control designs in the study of common diseases: updates on the demise of the rare disease assumption and the choice of sampling scheme for controls. *Int J Epidemiol* 1990; **19**: 205–13.

6 Some statistical procedures that are often used in epidemiology

Here we take a practically oriented look at some of the simple statistical methods and procedures that may be useful for preliminary analysis of data. The confidence interval for a proportion is described, and the t test is introduced. The χ^2 test is presented at some length, and Fisher's test gets a mention. Finally, some common misconceptions about significance testing are discussed.

This is not a statistics textbook, and a large number of very good medical statistic books exist. However, there are a number of simple statistical calculations that are quite often very useful in epidemiology, and most of which can be performed on a pocket calculator. It gives a certain feeling of self-confidence to be able to give an approximate confidence interval for data one has produced, or to be able to check the calculations in some published paper. This chapter just contains some statistical procedures that I myself often have found handy.

Two procedures have already been introduced in the previous chapters, namely how to calculate 95% confidence intervals for odds ratios and relative risks. This can be done quickly, and gives a sense of the possible ranges of the ORs and RRs, although you will find that for a surprising number of real studies the requirement that all cells of the 2×2 table must have a value of 10 or greater does not hold.

Another issue that is not uncommon in epidemiology is to estimate the confidence interval for a proportion.

Confidence intervals for proportions

Often, one wants to estimate the proportion of the population that have some characteristic, such as the proportion who have antibodies to disease A, or the proportion of the population who have had a test for disease B. It is seldom possible to test or ask everyone, so one would probably do this by collecting a random sample.

Assuming that this sample is truly random, with no selection biases involved, one would want to know how the proportion measured in the sample relates to the true prevalence in the population. This is exactly the same reasoning as we followed in Chapter 4 regarding the confidence interval for ORs: if one only wants to make a statement about the sample just studied there is no need for confidence intervals. If 31 subjects out of 100 tested had antibodies to hepatitis A, then seroprevalence in this group is 31%, and could not be otherwise. However, this is a very rare situation, and one usually wants the results to be applicable to some larger population.

One intuitively feels that the size of the sample is important. If three persons out of a sample of ten had antibodies to hepatitis A, then chance could play a major role. The 'true' seroprevalence in the population could easily have been closer to 20 or 40%, and one would hesitate to state that it was 30%. If however, we took a sample 100 subjects out of a large population and found 31 to be seropositive, we would feel more secure about the estimate of 'about 30%', and even more so if 308 out of 1,000 sampled were found to have antibodies. The larger the sample, the less influence will there be from the random inclusion of a couple of seropositives 'too many' or 'too few'.

The confidence interval for a proportion is calculated in the following fashion:

1. Write the number as a proportion instead as a percentage. For the last sample in the above paragraph the proportion would be 0.308 (308 persons out of 1,000 tested).
2. Call this proportion p. Call the total number of subjects in the study N.
3. Calculate the number $p \times (1 - p)/N$. In our example this would be $0.308 \times 0.692/1000$.
4. Immediately take the square root of this number

$$\sqrt{\frac{p \times (1-p)}{N}} \text{ or in the example } \sqrt{\frac{0.308 \times 0.692}{1000}} = 0.015$$

5. This number is called the *standard error of a proportion*.
6. Just as to get the error factor in the previous chapters, we now multiply the standard error by 2, and again this is a statistical device to create a 95% confidence interval:

$$2 \times 0.015 = 0.030$$

7. However, this time we do not divide and multiply by our final number, but instead subtract and add it to the original proportion (0.308 in the example):

Lower bound: $0.308 - 0.030 = 0.278$
Upper bound: $0.308 + 0.030 = 0.338$

8. In words: we assume that we have taken a truly random sample (no biases) of 1,000 people out of a much larger population. In this sample we have found 308 subjects to be positive for hepatitis A antibody. We can then state that with 95% probability the true seroprevalence in the population must be between 27.8% and 33.8%.

Observe the caveat about bias: if the sample was biased in some way, the calculated proportion will be false and the confidence interval will be meaningless. If we asked 1,000 people if they had had an HIV test, but several of those who had had a test said that they had not, then our calculated proportion for the total population would be too low, and this fact is in no way amended by adding a confidence interval to the figure. The confidence interval only shows the possible influence of chance (or *sampling error*) – it cannot be expected to read people's minds.

Significance testing

It is becoming more and more recognized by medical researchers and statisticians that the most informative way to indicate the statistical significance of a given value is to also present the confidence interval. In the examples for ORs and RRs in the previous chapters, two things are immediately obvious from a confidence interval:

1. If the 95% confidence interval does not include 1 (the entire interval is either above or below 1), then we know that there is a good probability that the risk factor studied is really associated with disease, and that this is not just a chance finding.
2. The width of the confidence interval gives a feeling for how precisely the OR or RR was measured in the study. If the 95% confidence interval for an RR was found to be from 1.3 to 15,

then we would not really know if this was a very important risk factor for the disease (high RR) or a relatively minor one.

However, much of medical literature still uses *significance tests* for these purposes, and there are in fact instances when confidence intervals are difficult to calculate when significance values can be attained quite easily.

The most common question behind all significance tests is probably the following: one has just observed a difference between two groups of patients (one of the groups having, e.g. higher haemoglobin values, higher number of women, lower attack rate, longer incubation times, etc.). Is this just something that happened by chance, or does this point to a real difference between the groups?

The statistical theory behind attempts to answer this question is quite complex in parts, and often in significance testing in real life situations it is uncertain that the necessary theoretical assumptions are met for such tests to be valid. Also, there is a good deal of philosophy involved as to what probabilities actually mean in this situation. We will refrain from going into such discussions, but just point out that for any variable measured on a group of people, there will be some kind of random variation between the subjects. The above question then becomes: is the difference observed between the groups just due to this variability, so that people who have a high value happened to end up in one group and people with a low value in the other? Or would it be very unlikely that chance could divide a homogeneous group of people into two so seemingly disparate groups?

There are basically two different situations possible:

1. We have measured the value of some continuous variable for all members in two groups. This could be their height, their haemoglobin value, their age, their temperature, etc. All these variables have in common that they can assume, at least in principle, any value on a continuous line. This is not strictly true, because we would probably record height in whole centimetres only, or temperature only in steps of 0.1°C, but theoretically they are continuous. For each of our two groups we could calculate an average value, and then compare them.

2. People are grouped into categories, such as exposed/unexposed, ill/healthy, men/women, older than/younger than, etc. We then look at our two groups of patients to see if there are any differences in the proportions exposed/unexposed, ill/healthy, men/women, etc. between them.

The *t* test

In the first situation above with continuous data, one uses something called (Student's) *t* test to decide if there is a statistically significant difference between the two groups. Most basic statistics programmes for a personal computer can do this very simply: one just enters the values for one of the patient groups in one column, and the values for the other group in the next column, and the programme delivers the probability (the *p value*) that chance alone would cause a difference between the two groups as big as or bigger than the actually observed one. The lower the *p* value, the less likely it is that this is a chance finding, and the more it is likely that there is a real difference between the groups.

The way to perform a *t* test is a follows:
1. Call the groups 1 and 2. The numbers of subjects in the groups are called n_1 and n_2 respectively.
2. The average value for the first group (e.g. of the haemoglobin values) is called m_1, and m_2 for the second group.
3. Calculate the standard deviation of the values in the two groups separately: for the first group, subtract m_1 from each of the values, square these differences, and add all the squares. Then divide this number by (n_1-1), and take the square root of this number. The resulting figure is the standard deviation of the values in group 1, and is called s_1. Written in mathematics:

$$s_1 = \sqrt{\sum_1^n \frac{(x_i - m_1)^2}{(n_1 - 1)}}$$

where x_i are all the individual measurements of the group. Then calculate s_2 in the same way.
The standard deviation is one way of describing how clustered the values in a group are around the average. A low standard deviation means that all the values are huddled close to the mean, a high standard deviation tells that they are spread widely.
4. One also needs a combined standard deviation for both groups. This is called s_p, and is calculated as

$$s_p^2 = \frac{(n_1 - 1)s_1^2 + (n_2 - 1)s_2^2}{n_1 + n_2 - 2}$$

5. The final figure we want is called *t*, and is defined as:

$$t = \frac{m_1 - m_2}{s_p \sqrt{1/n_1 + 1/n_2}}$$

6. This *t* value is then taken along to a ready-made table of *t*s, which is found at the back of most statistics textbooks. The actual significance levels vary with the sizes of the two groups, but as a general rule of thumb, a *t* value over about 2 means that there is a 5% chance or less that this difference between the two means would have arisen just by chance.

One can see that carrying out a t test becomes quite laborious even for rather small samples. One should use a computer for this, and the above points are included more to demonstrate how it is actually being done.

Two things are directly obvious, however. The higher the *t* value, the less probability that the observed difference in averages between the groups is just a chance finding. From the last formula it can be seen that the greater the difference between the means, the higher will the *t* value be. Also the smaller the combined measure of spread around the average values (s_p), the higher the *t* value will be. A small difference between two groups may be quite significant if the standard deviations are low, whereas a large difference between two groups with high standard deviations might just be a chance finding.

There is one restriction on the usage of the *t* test: if the standard deviations of the two groups are very different (say, one is more than twice as great as the other), then the *t* test should not be performed as described above. However, your favourite statistical computer programme may have a valid test for the occasion, or else consult a statistician, since very different spreads in the two groups may mean that you should be interested in more than just comparing the two means.

The Chi-squared (χ^2) test

In the second of the two situations above, we did not have continuous measurements of some variable for the two groups, but instead numbers of people belonging to different categories. It then becomes a bit strange to talk about the 'average sex' in a group of patients. The basic situation is just our familiar friend the 2×2 table, which could be for example:

	Vaccinated	Not vaccinated	
Ill	10	40	50
Well	80	20	100
	90	60	150

However, the 2 × 2 table could just as easily be extended to a table with more columns and/or rows if there were more categories of exposure or outcome or both.

In this situation, the subjects could only belong to the two categories 'vaccinated' or 'not vaccinated', and to either of the categories 'ill' or 'well'. There is no meaningful way of giving an average value of health in the vaccinated group, or an average vaccination status in the well group. This type of data is thus quite different from the *t* test situation above, and is usually called categorical as opposed to continuous data.

In Chapter 4 we saw how to calculate an OR for such a table, and also a confidence interval for this value. If we now want to perform a significance test instead, the question to ask is: what is the probability that the 150 subjects of the study would divide this way into 'ill' and 'well' just by chance? A very low probability of such a chance would give increased weight to our hypothesis that the vaccine has effect.

The way to reason is as follows: there are 50 people who fall ill and 100 who remain well. If the vaccine was totally inefficient, we would assume that it did not matter whether or not a subject was vaccinated. Since one third of the total group fall ill, this would be the expected proportion in each of the individual groups. In the vaccinated group of 90 people, we would expect 30 to fall ill, and in the unvaccinated group of 60, 20. The expected 2 × 2 table if the vaccine did not work at all would be:

Expected table	Vaccinated	Not vaccinated	
Ill	30	20	50
Well	60	40	100
	90	60	150

The general way of calculating the expected value for a cell in a 2 × 2 (or 3 × 3, or 5 × 3, or ...) table is to multiply the column sum at the bottom of the corresponding column by the row sum to the right, and dividing this number by the total in the lower right corner. For the first cell in our example this would be 90 × 50 / 150 = 30, just as above. (In these calculations, one often gets fractions of people in the cells of the expected table, but that does not affect the analysis at all.)

We can now compare the numbers in the expected table to the actual ones to see if they are very different. One way is to just take the difference between the numbers in the corresponding cells (10 − 30 for the first cell, 40 − 20 for the second, and so on). If the vaccine had no effect, we would expect those differences to be small, and the larger they are, the more the result of our study deviates from what would be expected just by chance distribution of the cases. The χ^2 test now consists of squaring all these differences, dividing each square by its expected value (from the table above), and then adding them. The higher this number, the less chance that the distribution of ill and healthy subjects according to vaccination status could have occurred just by chance. For a 2×2 table like this, a χ^2 value above 3.84 indicates that there is less than 5% probability that the result occurred by chance.

In the example above, the calculation would be:

$$\chi^2 = (10-30)^2/30 + (40-20)^2/20 + (80-60)^2/60 + (20-40)^2/40 = 50$$

We can see that there is a very small chance indeed that this high χ^2 value would arise by chance, and we can state that there is statistical support that the vaccine does have a protective effect. In fact, the probability that this would be a chance finding can be calculated to be $p < 0.0001$.

When you look up a χ^2 table, you will find that they mention something called 'degrees of freedom'. For tables such as the above, this has to do with the numbers of rows and columns (categories for exposure and outcome). The number of degrees of freedom is just (number of rows -1) $\times$ (number of columns -1), and thus for a 2×2 table $(2-1) \times (2-1) = 1$. For a 3×4 table (three different outcomes, four different exposures), there would be $(3-1) \times (4-1) = 6$ degrees of freedom, and you would have to refer to this table for the χ^2 test. (Degrees of freedom is often abbreviated 'd.f.')

A quick way to calculate the χ^2 value from the general 2×2 table from Chapter 4

	Exposed	**Not exposed**	
Cases	a	b	$a+b$
Controls	c	d	$c+d$
	$a+c$	$b+d$	N

is with the formula

$$\chi^2 = \frac{(ad-bc)^2 \times N}{(a+c)(b+d)(a+b)(c+d)}$$

where the parentheses in the denominator are just the column and row sums.

Since the χ^2 test is so easy to perform, it can often be used for an initial check even for continuous data, where one would otherwise use the *t* test. If one for example wants to compare temperatures in two groups of patients, one could just choose a value that seems to be somewhere in the middle of all temperature readings from both groups, and count the number of subjects in each group who have a temperature above or below this value. The four figures thus attained are entered into a 2×2 table, and the χ^2 calculated. If this χ^2 figure yields a low *p* value, then you can be quite confident that the *t* test will also yield a low *p* value.

There are, however, some important restrictions on when the χ^2 test can be used. It is an approximate method that gets more and more valid the larger the size of the study. As rules of thumb these restrictions are:

1. Either the total sample size (*N* above) should be greater than 40, or
2. *N* could be between 20 and 40, but none of the *expected* values in the 2×2 table should be smaller than 5.

If neither of these conditions are fulfilled, one must use Fisher's test, which is the subject of the next section.

Fisher's exact test

This test is a favourite with medical researchers, part of the explanation perhaps being the word 'exact' in the name of the test. It builds on the same general idea as the two tests above: what is the chance/probability that the pattern of outcomes we have observed would arise just by chance? Fisher's test is mostly used for 2×2 tables in which the individual values are too small for a χ^2 test to be allowed. If we have a 2×2 table looking like:

	Exposed	**Unexposed**	
Cases	8	2	10
Controls	3	5	8
	11	7	18

we cannot use the χ^2 test, nor can we use the formula for the confidence interval of an OR from Chapter 4. The concept behind Fisher's test is the following: in this study we had 10 cases and eight controls. Eleven subjects were exposed and seven were not exposed. These four figures make up the row and column sums, respectively. Keeping these row and column sums constant, in how many different ways could the 18 subjects of the study be distributed on the four different cells? Two other possibilities would be:

	Exposed	Not exposed				Exposed	Not exposed	
Cases	8	2	10	and	**Cases**	9	1	10
Controls	3	5	8		**Controls**	2	6	8
	11	7	18			11	7	18

and there are obviously several other distributions possible. The probability of getting any given 2 × 2 table when the row and column sums are fixed can be shown to be:

$$\frac{(a+c)!(b+d)!(a+b)!(c+d)!}{a!b!c!d!N!}$$

where a, b, c and d are the four cells as usual. The exclamation mark stands for 'factorial', and $a!$ is defined as multiplying a and all the integers less than a down to 1. The symbol 6! thus means $6 \times 5 \times 4 \times 3 \times 2 \times 1 = 720$. (By definition $0! = 1$.)

Using this formula, we can calculate the probability of getting the first 2 x 2 table of this section as

$$\frac{11!7!10!8!}{8!2!3!5!18!} = 0.08$$

However, we are not interested only in the probability of this distribution, but also in the chance to get an even more extreme result from a random spread of the 18 subjects. 'Extreme' here means an even greater difference in the proportion exposed among the cases and the controls. The second 2 × 2 table of the two alternatives above would thus be more extreme than our original one, and the most extreme distribution which would still conform with our fixed row and column totals would be

	Exposed	Unexposed	
Cases	10	0	10
Controls	1	7	8
	11	7	18

where there were no unexposed at all among the cases, and only one exposed among the eight controls.

In calculating the *p* value for a distribution of cases according to Fisher's test, we add the probability for the observed distribution to the probabilities for all more extreme distributions possible. In this example the probabilities for the two more extreme distributions can be calculated to be 0.009 and 0.0003, respectively, with the formula above. The *p* value would be 0.08 + 0.009 + 0.0003 = 0.081, and it would thus be quite likely that we would get the observed distribution at the top of this section just by chance.

Even for very low numbers in the 2 × 2 table, Fisher's test becomes very time consuming to perform, and the use of some standard statistics programme for a computer is strongly recommended.

One-sided and two-sided testing

An additional issue in significance testing concerns whether one should make so-called one-sided or two-sided tests. This is again a somewhat philosophical discussion, and really depends on the assumptions one makes before performing the test. The basic hypothesis (often called *the null hypothesis*) in the three statistical methods described above is always that there is no real difference between the groups, and that the observed difference is a random effect. We then proceed to calculate the probability that this difference would arise just at random, and if this probability is very small, we deduce that it is unlikely that we have made a chance finding.

If we have no *a priori* idea about which direction the difference between the groups may go, i.e. that it is just as plausible that the average temperature in group A will be higher than in group B as the other way around, then we should perform a two-sided test. This will tell us the added probabilities of observing as high, or higher, a difference in mean temperature A − B and of observing the same difference B − A.

If, however, we have some previous knowledge that treatment C is at least as good as treatment D, and possibly better, then we are only interested in finding out if the patients receiving C fare significantly better than those on D. In this instance we could make a one-sided test of significance, which would tell us the probability that the C patients fared as well or better compared with the D patients just by chance.

The χ^2 test is always two-sided and does thus not differ between the ways in which the observed difference may go. Tables for the *t* test include columns for both one-sided and two-sided tests, whereas Fisher's test as described above is one-sided. One simple approximation to make the p value given by Fisher's test apply to a two-sided situation is to just double it.

It may be tempting to choose the p value for the one-sided test from a t table, since it is always lower than the two-sided one, but this can only be done if one has firm prior knowledge that the observed difference can only go in one direction. In a test of a new drug, it would be just as important to find out that it was actually detrimental to the patients as that it was beneficial, and our test must include both these possibilities.

General notes on significance tests

Like all the concepts borrowed into epidemiology from statistical theory, significance tests assume unbiased sampling. A p value only tells us the probability that the difference we have observed is due to chance and random effects. If there was a bias in the selection of subjects, or in the type of exposure between the groups, or in the measurement of outcomes, the p value will tell us nothing about the precision or validity of our findings.

There are two common misconceptions in the interpretation of p values. The first assumes that a low, or very low, p value 'proves' that the difference we have found is due to the treatment, or to the exposure, etc. Statistical hypothesis testing by significance analysis never proves anything, it just tells us that the probability that our observed effect should be due to chance is low. If one wants to be very careful, one should thus state the findings as: 'Statistical significance testing gives an indication that the observed finding is not just due to chance.'

Continuing this line of reasoning, one should remember that many articles in medical literature regard a p value of less than 5% as significant. This is equivalent to stating that there is only one chance in 20 that the result was due to chance. Strictly interpreted, this means that out of 20 such studies reporting significant associations, 1 will just be a chance finding. With the large volume of scientific medical articles being published each month, the number that report spurious findings as facts is thus hardly negligible.

The second misconception works in the opposite way. If the outcome of a study was found not to be statistically significant, this is sometimes reported as 'there is no association between exposure A and outcome B'. This may be completely wrong, and there may be quite a strong association, although the study failed to confirm it.

Mostly, this is due to too small sample size, and a similar study on a larger number of subjects may well reveal significant differences. A lack of significance in a test does not prove that the opposite is true.

Finally, just a paragraph about the word 'significance'. This is a word with many positive connotations, but one should always remember that it only addresses statistical significance. A very significant statistical finding may have a very low clinical significance. Studies may show a significantly increased risk of developing Hodgkin's disease after tonsillectomy in puberty, but the risk to the individual is so small anyway that even a doubling may be personally insignificant, since the vast majority of people who have had a tonsillectomy will not develop this lymphoma. Not even for differential diagnosis in patients with prolonged fever will the fact that the patient has had a tonsillectomy give much assistance. The clinical significance of such a finding would be low.

Summary

If we study a sample of subjects from a larger population, there will always be a chance component as to which subjects we happened to choose. We may have happened to include too many subjects with disease A, or too few with antibody to disease B. Statistical theory tells us how different our sample is likely to be from the total population and expresses this by assigning confidence intervals to figures estimated from the sample that tell us which values are likely for these figures in the total population.

If we find a large difference between two study groups, either in some continuous variable such as haemoglobin value or age, or in the proportion of subjects with different characteristics, we could calculate the probability that the difference would have arisen by chance. For continuous variables this is done with the t test, for categorical with the χ^2 test. If the numbers of a 2×2 table are small, Fisher's test gives a better alternative to χ^2 tests.

As a rule of thumb, a t value greater than 2, and a χ^2 value for a 2×2 table greater than 4 indicate that the finding is statistically significant on the 5% level.

A finding that statistically is very significant could well be of little clinical significance.

7 Clinical epidemiology: sensitivity, specificity, misclassification

Here we discuss how well we measure the things we want to study. A test is characterized by its sensitivity and specificity, but one also has to consider the context in which it will be used. When measurement is imprecise, we will place subjects in the wrong groups, which is called misclassification, and might have serious consequences.

Sensitivity and specificity

In order to make a diagnosis, we interview the patient, we make a physical examination, and we may perform tests or investigations. For each of these steps certain findings will indicate that the patient has a certain disease – with greater or lesser probability. Likewise, we know that the absence of certain findings might indicate that the patient does not have the disease. The two main terms used to describe how well a test performs are *sensitivity* and *specificity*. These two terms are not very fortunate, partly because they are too similar and partly because they do not give any intuitive feeling for what they mean.

Sensitivity measures how often a test turns out positive when it is being used on people that we (in some other way) know to have the disease. If one, for example, takes a cervical chlamydial sample for culture from 100 women with chlamydia infection, the culture will be positive in 80 of them at most – the test method is simply not perfect. In this case we say that the sensitivity of chlamydia culture is 80%.

Another example is culture of stools for salmonella. In asymptomatic carriers, the sensitivity of one faecal culture is only around 70%. By taking a second sample, we will get a positive culture from some of those who were negative the first time, and by taking a third sample we may find salmonella in some of the remainders. By counting all the people who have at least one positive culture, sensitivity could be raised to over 90%. This is the reason for using repeated cultures when looking for salmonella carriers.

An example of a test with low sensitivity is blood culture from patients with agranulocytosis and suspect bacteraemia. Pathogens are seldom found, but in most cases one never the less chooses to treat with antibiotics just on the suspicion of bacteraemia.

Observe that the definition of sensitivity implies that there is a *gold standard* (or 'truth') somewhere: there must be another way to decide unambiguously whether the patient has the disease or not. As you are surely aware, there are not many diseases for which this is true, and sensitivity is thus a somewhat abstract measure. Most often, sensitivity is actually being measured against the best available previous test.

Specificity is rather the reverse: it tells how often the test turns out negative when it is being used on people that we know do *not* have the disease. Ideally, a test for a disease should always be negative when used on healthy people, and such a test would be said to have a 100% specificity. An example: before it became possible to test for infection with hepatitis C in presumptive blood donors, some blood banks used a raised alanine-amino-transferase (ALT) value as marker of possible hepatitis. However, if this test was applied to a large group of donors, there would among them be several who had elevated ALT-values for other reasons, but who would be excluded from donating blood because they would be suspected to have hepatitis. This particular test would have a specificity well below 100% in the diagnosis of hepatitis. This lack of specificity may not be a great problem for the blood bank, because other donors could be found, but it may create problems for the excluded donors who were told that they might have an infectious hepatitis.

Low sensitivity means that the test will miss a lot of people who have the disease, whilst low specificity implies that the test will put many people in the 'disease group' who do not have the disease. In epidemiological jargon, one often says that a test with poor sensitivity will give raise to a lot of 'false negatives', whereas one with poor specificity will yield a lot of 'false positives'.

Few tests used in medicine have a specificity over 99%, but an example of the importance of high specificity comes from the use of HIV tests: if we tested 500,000 blood donors for HIV infection each year with an antibody test having 'only' 99% specificity, we would label 5,000 positive, even if there were not one single case of 'true' HIV infection in the group. In reality, things are not that bad: the specificity of the present HIV antibody tests is only some tenths of a percent below 100%, and all positive results are verified with Western blots, which means that the problem with false positives is negligible.

An example of a test with low specificity is the use of nasopharyngeal culture to decide whether or not a child with a runny nose should have antibiotics. Many children carry *Haemophilus influenza* or *Branhamella catarrhalis* behind their noses without needing any treatment with antibiotics, and the result of the test would not guide our decision very much.

For most tests there is a conflict between demands for high sensitivity and high specificity. A good example comes from the use of serology to decide whether or not a patient has had an infection: for such a test one needs a cut-off point at a certain antibody titre, so that those who have higher values will be said to have had the disease in question, whereas those with lower titres are said not to have had it. If this cut-off value is set very low, one will not miss any of those with past infection (high sensitivity), but one will also include a number of persons who only have unspecific reactions to the test, without any real markers (low specificity). If one instead raises the cut-off point, one will not call anyone with unspecific reaction positive (high specificity), but instead miss a number of patients who have true low levels of markers of past infection (low sensitivity). We will return to the question of cut-off points in Chapter 15 on serology.

While the words sensitivity and specificity are most often employed in connection with laboratory tests, it is quite useful to think in those terms even about the interview or physical examination. The presence of Koplik's spots on the inside of the cheek in a child diagnoses measles with a very high specificity (it cannot be anything else), whereas cough in the same child diagnoses measles with a very high sensitivity ('Without cough, no measles' as my old professor used to say – even if this criterion will also include lots of children who do not have measles which equals low specificity).

It is also worthwhile to ponder the high diagnostic specificity of the first moments of your contact with a patient. An unknown patient waiting outside your office door could have anyone of thousands of diseases. As soon as he/she comes in the door, at least 50% of these become implausible: you see the gender, the approximate age, the gait, the general appearance. After the first minute of talking, you are probably down to at most 10 possible diagnoses.

We seldom pause to think about the enormous speed at which this diagnostic process runs, excluding 99% of all diagnoses in next to no time, and leaving a very small number for more elaborate tests and procedures. It could be described as a chain of unconscious 'tests', where we confidently exclude diagnoses with a very high specificity.

An example

A study from Malawi attempted to assess the sensitivity and specificity of directly observable clinical signs for the diagnosis of malaria and pneumonia in children:[1]

The study subjects were 1,469 children under five years of age who came to a children's outpatient department with fever and/or cough. The purely clinical definition of malaria was:

* fever or history of fever

and the definition of pneumonia was:

* history of cough, or
* difficulty in breathing and lower chest-wall indrawing, or
* increased respiratory rate.

Blood films for microscopic examination for malaria parasites were taken from all children, but only those with evidence of pneumonia (or who had parasitaemia) had a chest X-ray.

A total of 1,290 children fulfilled the clinical definition for malaria. Of these, 486 had a positive blood film, whilst in 804 no parasitaemia could be diagnosed. One hundred and seventy-nine children did not meet the clinical case definition, but of these 22 had a positive blood film.

If we assume that 'positive blood film' is the gold standard for diagnosing malaria, we would say that our clinical case definition has correctly diagnosed 486 out of all the 486 + 22 = 508, truly infected children. The sensitivity of the clinical definition will thus be:

$$\text{Sensitivity} = \frac{486}{508} = 96\%$$

which means that out of all the truly infected this crude "test" will identify almost everyone.

On the other hand, only 157 of the malaria-negative children were correctly labelled negative by the clinical definition. There were also 804 who were initially judged to be positive, but who were negative in their blood films. The total number of true negatives was thus 804 + 157 = 961, and the specificity of the clinical definition becomes

$$\text{Specificity} = \frac{157}{961} = 16\%$$

which means that five out of six children who did not have malaria would still be diagnosed as having the disease by the clinical definition.

Stated in words, what we have found is that almost all cases of malaria will have or have had fever, but that many cases of fever will not be malaria.

Since children without clinical symptoms of pneumonia were not X-rayed, we have no 'gold standard' for this disease and cannot calculate the sensitivity or specificity of these three clinical signs for the diagnosis of pneumonia.

Positive predictive value

This is a very important concept, which is frequently overlooked when merits of different tests are discussed. It has to do with the environment in which the test is being used – the same test might be useful in one setting and have a limited value in another. Whereas a test for haematuria might diagnose schistosomiasis infection with high probability in a region in Africa, it would not serve this purpose in Europe, where the prevalence of this infection is low, and most cases of haematuria are due to other causes.

If a test has 100% sensitivity and 100% specificity it does not matter where one uses it; it will correctly label everybody tested anyway. However, when these values (as they always do) lie below 100%, the actual prevalence of the disease one is testing for becomes important. The problem arises from the way one should interpret a result of the test.

Let us assume that we have an HIV antibody test with 99.9% sensitivity and 99.5% specificity and that we do not have access to Western blot. We want to use it to determine the HIV prevalence in a population of 10,000, where the true prevalence (which is unknown to us, but has been ascertained in some mysterious way) is 10%.

There must thus be 1,000 seropositive persons in this population, and since our test has 99.9 sensitivity, it will correctly label 999 of these as being infected. One infected will not be diagnosed. There are also 9,000 seronegative persons, and with the given specificity, $0.995 \times 9,000 = 8,955$ of these will be labelled as being negative. However, our test will also yield 45 false positives.

The *positive predictive value* (PPV) is the proportion of all test-positives who really are infected. In this case $999 + 45 = 1,044$ will have a positive test, but we know that only 999 of those are really infected:

$$\text{PPV} = \frac{999}{999 + 45} = \frac{999}{1044} = 0.957, \text{ or } 96\%$$

This means that for someone with a positive test, there is a 96% probability that he really is infected, which explains the term positive predictive value.

Now let us use the same test in another population of 10,000 subjects, where the true (equally mysteriously assessed) prevalence is 1/1,000:

There are thus 10 seropositive individuals, and our test will correctly identify all of them. There are also 9,990 seronegative persons, and of these $0.995 \times 9,990 = 9,940$ will have a negative test result. However, 50 will be false positives. In this case the positive predictive value will be

$$\text{PPV} = \frac{10}{10 + 50} = \frac{10}{60} = 0.166, \text{ or } 17\%$$

In this second population, a person who tests positive will thus have only a 17% chance of being truly infected, whereas 83% of those that the test calls positive are in reality seronegative. It is clear that even this exceedingly good test becomes quite useless in this population.

(One might argue that it is not much more fun to be mislabelled positive in a high-prevalence than in a low-prevalence population, and that the number of false positives is about equal in the two cases. This is a valid point, but for diagnostic purposes, and even more so for epidemiology, there is a large difference in the applicability of the test in the two situations. If you were to give someone treatment on the results of only one test like this, you would feel a lot better if you knew that there was a high chance that he really had the disease.)

The simplest way to think about the PPV is to look at the specificity of the test, and see what percentage of the population will be false positive. This number will be the same in all populations, regardless of the true prevalence. One then considers the expected prevalence, to see if it is considerably higher than the false positive portion. If it is, one can disregard the false positives, and the test will be useful. This simplified way of looking at PPV comes from the fact that most laboratory tests have a sensitivity of at least 90%, and then the specificity becomes much more crucial for the PPV.

In the malaria example above, the PPV for the clinical definition would have been $486/1290 = 38\%$. Obviously, this value would have been even lower in a setting where malaria was less common.

When a new test has been developed, its sensitivity and specificity have often been measured under very ideal circumstances, with much attention paid to technical detail, and a high-prevalent group of samples for evaluation. As the test enters clinical medicine, it often performs worse. This is due to a number of factors, from less experienced staff to lower overall prevalence in the population tested.

A new 2 × 2 table

All the above terms can be nicely defined using our old friend, the 2 × 2 table. It looks like before, but the rows and columns are named differently:

	Test positive	Test negative	
Have disease	a	b	$a + b$
Healthy	c	d	$c + d$
	$a + c$	$b + d$	

In a perfect test, c and b are both $= 0$, since only those who are ill test positive and only those who are healthy test negative.

The definitions of our terms are:

$$\text{Sensitivity} = \frac{a}{a + b}$$

$$\text{Specificity} = \frac{d}{c + d}$$

$$\text{PPV} = \frac{a}{a + c}$$

and there is also a thing called *negative predictive value* (NPV), defined as

$$\text{NPV} = \frac{d}{b + d}$$

which is the reverse of the PPV, i.e. the proportion truly healthy out of all those with a negative test.

Personally, I always find all these definitions impossible to remember, and I have to look them up every time I need them. It might be a good idea for you to fold the top corner of this page ('a dog's ear'), so that you will know where to look for this schematic 2×2 table in the future.

As pointed out above, we should probably be thinking more in terms of sensitivity and specificity for the questions we use when we interview a patient, or the physical examinations we perform. There is a lot of historical deadwood here, and much of it arguably adds very little to the diagnostic process.

Reliability

This term describes how 'constant' a test is, i.e. will it give the same value if used repeatedly on the same sample? We would not want it to come out with different answers at different times. Also, will the test yield the same result in different laboratories? Another term is that the test should be *reproducible*. High reliability is mostly a problem for the laboratory people, but even when clinical measurements are concerned, reliability can be improved by letting several independent doctors judge a specific finding.

Validity

This is a more subtle concept than reliability, and has to do with the question whether we really measure what we want to know. Using the presence or absence of a high sedimentation rate to decide which patients have a bacterial infection, and should be given antibiotics, is not a very valid test.

A test may be perfectly reliable, giving quite dependable values each time, but still not tell us what we want to know about the patient's disease. If the association between test result and 'true' disease in the patient is weak, then this test would not be very valid for the situation in which we apply it.

Misclassification

In the discussions of risks, RRs, ORs and rate ratios of the previous chapters, we assumed that all study subjects were assigned to the correct groups, whether it be what they were exposed to or what happened to them.

One exception is from the very first example in Chapter 3, where one of the guests at the dinner could have forgotten what he ate (uncertain exposure). Another was in the discussion of biases in connection with the person-year graph in Chapter 5, where it was pointed out that if the subjects that we designed as 'losses to follow-up' really had died (uncertain outcome), this would underestimate the rate.

It has been said that good epidemiology really is a question of accurate measurements. If the subjects are somehow classified in the wrong group, this is called *misclassification*. There are two types, random and nonrandom mis-classification.

Random misclassification

This is the lesser of the two problems. It appears when our methods of measuring risk factors or disease are less than perfect, as they almost always are. Let us look at an example:[2]

In a case-control study in Gothenburg, 5,741 young women were tested for chlamydia infection, and at the same time asked about certain risk factors for being infected. One such 'risk factor' studied was the duration of their present sexual relationship. The women who had no partner or whose present relationship had lasted less than one year were compared to those who had a steady sexual partner for more than one year. The actual 2×2 table for this factor was

	Present relationship ≤ 1 year	**Present relationship > 1 year**	
Chlamydia positive	280	144	424
Chlamydia negative	2408	2909	5317
	2688	3053	5741

From this table we can see that the OR for being infected if the present relationship had lasted less than one year was $(280/2408)/(144/2909) = 2.35$. There thus seems to be lower risk of being infected with chlamydia if one has a longer, steady relationship, which seems plausible.

However, we learnt from the discussion about sensitivity above that a chlamydia culture only correctly identifies 80% of the infected. This means that we have missed 20% of the infected. The true total number of infected should not have been 424 as in the 2×2 table, but 25% more, or 530. How should these extra 106 cases be divided on the two groups of women?

Obviously, there must be equal chance of being a false negative whether one has had a short relationship or a long one: the length of the relation can hardly affect the sensitivity of the test. This is just what we mean by random misclassification, it affects both groups in the same way. Thus, the number of infected in both groups should really increase by 25%. In the short relationship group, 25% × 280 = 70, more of those labelled negative should have been positive, and in the long relationship group, 25% × 180 = 36 truly positive were not diagnosed.

The specificity of a chlamydia culture is 100% for all practical purposes, so there are no false positives. The 'true' 2 × 2 table would thus have been

	Present relationship ≤ 1 year	Present relationship > 1 year	
Chlamydia positive	350	180	530
Chlamydia negative	2338	2873	5211
	2688	3053	5741

where we have added 70 positives to the short relationship group (and taken away 70 negatives), and moved 36 women from the negative square to the positive in the long relationship group.

The OR for this table would be (350/2338)/(180/2873) = 2.39, or slightly higher than the value 2.35 above. This difference may not be very impressive, but the exercise points to the main feature of random misclassification: *it lessens the strength of the associations found in an epidemiological study*. This means that random misclassification will never create a bias that makes a factor seem significant for development of disease, but it may well lessen the true value of an OR or an RR so that they no longer seem to be significant. In our example, the less than total sensitivity of the test for chlamydia makes the OR seem slightly lower than it should have been.

This misclassification was about disease versus no disease, but the same reasoning applies if exposure had been randomly misclassified. In this example exposure could have been misclassified if for example some proportion of the women who reported long relationships really had had short ones and vice versa. Such random misclassification would also have rendered the OR too low.

Nonrandom (or preferential) misclassification

This is a much worse problem, and a bias introduced by nonrandom misclassification could really go any way. It occurs when for example the test we use behaves differently in the different groups we are studying. A simple, constructed example would be the following: imagine that we wanted to find out if patients presenting with a sore throat would be more likely to have infectious mononucleosis if they were adolescents than if they were children, and that we would base the diagnosis on the Monospot test. The sensitivity of this test is good for ages round puberty, but low in small children, which means that we would selectively miss a part of the children with infectious mononucleosis. Such a study could thus lead to the result that infectious mononucleosis was a more common cause of sore throat in adolescents, even if this were false.

Nonrandom misclassification is really just another name for the different types of biases discussed at the end of Chapter 5, and just like these, it can often be eliminated by careful clinical consideration.

Summary

Epidemiology is very much about good measurements. If the outcome of a study is whether or not the patient dies, or if the risk factor studied is gender, this is usually a small problem, but as soon as we use some kind of test to measure exposure or outcome, bias might be introduced.

The ability of a test to pick out the truly diseased in a population is called sensitivity, whereas its ability to select the healthy ones is called specificity.

The usefulness of a test depends not only on these two numbers, but also on the prevalence of the disease in the population, and the three together define the positive predictive value.

Random misclassification can weaken an association, even to the point where a significant difference becomes insignificant, but can never create significant findings. Preferential misclassification is just another name for bias, and might work in any way in a study; nonsignificant associations becoming significant, and vice versa.

References

1. Redd SC, Bloland PB, Kazembe PN, Patrick E, Tembenu R, Campbell CC. Usefulness of clinical case-definition in guiding therapy for African children with malaria or pneumonia. *Lancet* 1992; **340**: 1140–43.

2. Ramstedt K, Forssman L, Giesecke J, Granath F. Risk factors for *Chlamydia trachomatis* infection in 6810 young women attending family planning clinics. *Int J STD & AIDS* 1992; **3**: 117–22.

8 Multivariate analysis and interaction

This discusses the simultaneous analysis of several risk factors. The procedure of stratification is explained, and the Mantel–Haenszel algorithm for calculating an adjusted RR or OR is described. The ideas behind matching receive a mention and the 2 × 2 table for matched studies is demonstrated. There is also a short introduction to the concept of regression models, and finally, interaction is discussed and exemplified.

Most of the examples given so far have only looked at one exposure and one outcome: type of food eaten versus risk for gastroenteritis in Chapter 3, HIV status and risk of tuberculosis in Chapter 5, or length of the relationship versus risk for chlamydia infection in the previous chapter. In many instances there may be several factors that are potentially associated with risk for disease. There are two different possibilities here:

1. Either we want to describe the independent contributions to risk for disease from several factors. Risk for infection with measles in a cohort of children could depend on family size, age, vaccination status, type of schooling, etc. Each of these factors could well play an independent role for the number of measles cases in the cohort during one year, and we may want to analyse them all.

2. Or, we just want to study the risk associated with one single factor. In the measles example, we could for example be interested in the association between age at vaccination and subsequent risk of measles infection. All the other variables, like family size, etc., would then just be potential confounders, and we would want to get rid of their influences in our calculation of an RR or OR.

From the point of view of the statistical analysis, it does not really matter which approach we choose. Statistics just measures the degree of association between any factor and disease, and is quite blind to the issue of causation or confounding. The decision to either regard the different variables as independently important or to regard one as primarily important and the others as confounders rests with the person performing the analysis, and also depends on the exact question being asked.

Adjusting for confounding

However, in many situations one is quite determined to study just one single risk factor for disease, and potential confounding effects from other factors should be eliminated as far as possible. In Chapter 4, it was mentioned that confounding can be adjusted for in the analysis, if only data on the confounding variable has been collected. The simplest way to grasp this is described below:

Confounding arises when the two groups one is comparing are not equal in some other real risk factor for the disease (other than the factor one wants to study, that is). If only the two groups were equal: same age distribution, same proportion of women, same nutritional status, etc., there would be no confounding. One way to solve this is to compare *subgroups* in which the subjects have similar values for the confounding variable, instead of making the comparison between the total of the two original groups. The results of these subgroup comparisons are then averaged in a clever fashion to give an overall RR or OR. These subgroups of subjects who have similar values for a confounder are often called *strata*, and the procedure called *stratification*. The resulting OR or RR is called *adjusted*, and by doing a stratified analysis, we have *controlled* for this confounder.

For example, a study wanted to see if the seroprevalence of antibody to infection with herpes simplex virus type 2 (HSV-2) was increasing over time in the population. This disease is mainly spread through sexual intercourse, and the seroprevalence has been suggested to be a good marker of sexual behaviour. Previous studies have shown that the risk of having markers for HSV-2 infection increases with the number of sexual partners a person has had in his/her life.

In order to do this, two random samples of pregnant women in Stockholm were tested for antibody: one group of 940 women who were pregnant in 1969, and another of 1,000 women pregnant in 1989. The seroprevalence in those two years was found to be 17 and

33%. For the purpose of this example, we will call the prevalence in 1969 baseline prevalence, and thus make the women of 1969 our comparison group. The risk ratio for being HSV-2 positive in 1989 compared to 1969 would be $0.33/0.17 = 1.9$.

Further analysis showed that in both groups of women, there was an increase in seroprevalence with age. When we hear this we should stop and ask ourselves: is there any other possible difference between the two groups, other than that they were pregnant 20 years apart? What happens if the women in one of the groups were older on average? Since age is associated with prevalence, this fact would by itself make prevalence higher in that group.

In effect, it was found that the mothers-to-be of 1989 were on average 4.4 years older than those of 1969: as in most industrialized countries women's age at the birth of their first child (and thus also of subsequent children) has increased in Sweden during the last decades. This is a nice example of confounding, since the two groups of women differed not only in year of pregnancy (which is the factor we want to study), but also in that the risk factor 'age' was not equally distributed among the two groups.

The way to control for age is to divide the women from both years into strata, where each *stratum* only contains women from a certain age group. The first stratum consists of the 1969 women who were 25 years or younger at the time of pregnancy, and of the 1989 women who were also 25 or younger at the time of their pregnancies. The second stratum contains the women aged 26-30 from both groups, and so on. The relative risk for infection in the 1989 women is then calculated within each stratum only (i.e. only for women of approximately the same age) (Table 8.1).

For each age group, the RR is calculated by dividing the seroprevalence in 1989 by the seroprevalence in 1969. You can see that in all but the youngest age groups ('strata'), the RR is lower than the overall RR in the bottom row. If you look closely at the number tested in each age group you can also see the reason for this: the average age of the women in 1989 was higher – there were for example 134 women out of 1,000 being older than 35 in 1989 versus only 26 out of 940 in 1969. Since prevalence was found to increase with age, this difference in age distribution will by itself lead to higher average prevalence in the women of 1989.

If we want to have one single figure to describe the increased risk of being HSV-2-positive in 1989, we need to adjust for this age difference. One way of doing this would be to just average the RRs for

Table 8.1 *Prevalence of antibody to herpes simplex virus type 2 by age group in samples of women in Stockholm pregnant in 1969 and 1989. The relative risks (RRs) for infection in 1989 are calculated setting the risk in 1969 to 1 for each age group*

Age group	1969			1989			RR
	Sero-Positive	Number tested	% positive	Sero-positive	Number tested	% positive	
up to 25	97	584	16.6	81	255	31.8	1.92
26–30	44	252	17.5	106	352	30.1	1.72
31–35	16	78	20.5	101	259	39.0	1.90
36 or older	6	26	23.1	42	134	31.3	1.35
Total	163	940	17.3	330	1000	33.0	1.91

the four age groups. However, the total numbers of women in the four age groups are rather different. Referring to the discussion about confidence intervals for proportions in Chapter 6, one would be more confident about the figure for seroprevalence in the women aged less than 25 in 1969, which is calculated as 97 positive out of 584 tested, than about the figure for women aged over 35 in 1969, which was based on only 26 women, six of whom were positive.

This intuition is supported by calculating the confidence intervals for each of the RRs. We again use the formula

$$\text{Error factor} = e^{2\times\sqrt{1/a+1/b}}$$

where a is number of positive women in 1969, and b is number of positives in 1989. Each RR is then divided and multiplied by its error factor to get an upper and lower bond. (You will notice that for the last RR this is not quite permitted, since one really needs at least 10 cases in each group, but we will disregard that here.)

The corresponding confidence intervals are given in Table 8.2. It is evident that the group with the least number of cases has the widest confidence interval.

Table 8.2 *Confidence intervals for the relative risks (RRs) for the study given in Table 8.1*

Age group	RR	95% confidence interval
–25	1.92	1.50 – 2.71
26–30	1.72	1.20 – 2.46
31–35	1.90	1.11 – 3.25
36–	1.35	0.56 – 3.23

The following description of Mantel–Haenszel weighted ratios is a bit technical, and you might be satisfied just knowing that an adjusted risk ratio can be calculated. I shall include it anyway for future reference. Should you ever want to calculate an adjusted RR or OR, the text below shows you how to do it.

If one wants to average the ratios properly, one should not take the plain average of the four numbers, but rather give them different weights, depending on how reliable each of the four RRs are. In this context 'reliable' is taken to mean the same as 'having a narrow confidence interval'. The narrower the confidence interval, the more credible is the RR, and the higher weight it gets. The best way to do that is to use a scheme described by Mantel and Haenszel, where each subgroup RR gets a weight in the following way:

1. Take the number of cases in the baseline, or *unexposed*, group (women pregnant in 1969 in this case). If we use the age group 26–30 as an example, this number would be 44.
2. Multiply by the total number of persons in the *exposed* group (which here would be the 1989 women). There were 352 women in the age group 26–30 in 1989.
3. Divide by the total number of individuals in that age group, adding the 1969 and the 1989 women. This would be $252 + 352 = 604$ for the age group 26–30.
4. The resulting figure is the Mantel–Haenszel weight of the RR for women in that age group: $44 \times 352 / (252 + 352) = 25.6$.

For all the age groups, the Mantel–Haenszel weights would be:

$$-25: \qquad w_{-25} = 97 \times 255 / (584 + 255) = 29.5$$

$$26 - 30: \qquad w_{25-30} = 44 \times 352 / (252 + 352) = 25.6$$

$$30 - 35: \qquad w_{30-35} = 16 \times 259 / (78 + 259) \ = 12.3$$

$$36-: \qquad w_{36-} = 6 \times 134 / (26 + 134) \ \ = 5.0$$

We see that the weight is highest for the group in which we have most data, and lowest where the number of women (and seropositive women) is lowest.

5. Each of the RRs is then multiplied by its corresponding weight and the four products are added.
6. This number is divided by the sum of all the weights. The final resulting number is the Mantel–Haenszel estimate of the adjusted RR:

$$RR_{MH} = \frac{(1.92 \times 29.5) + (1.72 \times 25.6) + (1.90 \times 12.3) + (1.35 \times 5.0)}{29.5 + 25.6 + 12.3 + 5.0} = 1.82$$

This adjustment procedure has thus lowered the estimated RR from a *crude* value of 1.91 in the table above to an *adjusted* value of 1.82. What we have done is to recognize that the 1989 women were older on average, and by calculating an RR_{MH}, we have effectively erased the effect of this confounder.

A point on words here: 'Adjusted' sounds impressive, and one immediately senses that an adjusted RR must be much better than a crude one, maybe it is even the 'true' RR. Just remember, once again, that we can only adjust for the confounders that we are aware of, and for which we have data. If there exist unknown confounders of the study, that have not been taken into account, no elaborate M–H weighting scheme is able to adjust for them. 'Adjusted' means adjusted for the confounders that we were able to imagine and measure, nothing else.

This was an example of a cross-sectional study, where risks and RRs could be calculated. If we are trying to adjust an OR from a case-control study for confounding, this can be done in exactly the same way, by calculating an OR for each stratum. The weights for these ORs are then calculated in the same way, but points 1–3 above would instead read:

Make a separate 2×2 table for each stratum. Then for each table:
1. Take the number of unexposed cases. (If you look back at the general 2×2 table of Chapter 4, this would correspond to *b*.)
2. Multiply by the number of exposed controls (*c* of the general 2×2 table).
3. Divide by the total number of individuals in that stratum ($ = a + b + c + d$).

This gives you the weight of the OR for this stratum, and they are then added as in points 5 and 6 above, to give an adjusted $OR_{MH.}$

In our study of pregnant women, it does seem that there had been a real increase in the risk of being infected with HSV-2 between 1969 and 1989, which could indicate that the latter group of women had had a higher number of partners on average before the blood sample was taken in connection with a pregnancy. Another possible explanation is that prevalence had increased in men during the 20-year period, so that the risk of becoming infected by any single partner had increased.

Just another point about confounding: a confounder is not something that is inherent to the data one is looking at. As was pointed out in Chapter 4, it is also a question of perspective. In the example above, we wanted to use seroprevalence of antibody to HSV-2 as a measure of changes in sexual behaviour between 1969 and 1989, which meant that we had to adjust for the age difference. Another side of HSV-2 infection is that it can be transmitted from mother to child during delivery and cause a serious disease in the newborn. An equally important question could therefore have been: 'What was the risk for a baby being born in 1989 compared with 1969 of having a mother who was seropositive for HSV-2?'. The answer to this question would be the crude risk ratio of 1.91, since the average risk to all babies would have nothing to do with the mothers' age distribution in the different years.

Matching

There is another, rather obvious, way to control for possible confounders already at the stage of data collection, and that is to *match* controls to the cases. Confounding arises when there is an imbalance between the groups regarding some risk factor for disease other than the one we want to study. Or put in another way: when comparing some outcome (e.g. attack rate) in two different groups, we want them to be as similar as possible in all respects, except for the factor we want to study (e.g. vaccination status). One way to do this is in a case-control study is to select controls that are similar to the cases regarding all the suspected confounders, such as age, sex, family size, school attended, etc. If we succeed in this, we will have controlled for these confounders in the study proper, and need not concern ourselves with the stratification methods above, or the regression methods below.

The analysis of a matched study becomes slightly different from a nonmatched study. We will not compare all the cases to all the controls, but rather analyse the differences within each matched pair. If we for example wanted to study the association between 'being a health care worker' and 'having markers of hepatitis B infection', we could select a group of health-care workers, choose a control for each person of same sex and age, and test the members of each pair for hepatitis B markers.

The result could be presented in a slightly modified 2 × 2 table like that on the next page.

This table shows that we have studied 150 pairs (150 health-care workers matched to 150 controls). In 100 of these pairs, both subjects had the same hepatitis B status: in 10 pairs both positive and in 90 pairs both negative. These pairs add nothing to our analysis, and are disregarded.

		Control:		
		Positive for markers	**Negative for markers**	
	positive for markers	10	30	40
Health-care worker:	**negative for markers**	20	90	110
		30	120	150

The interesting cells are the upper right-hand and the lower left-hand, in which the pairs are *discordant* regarding hepatitis B status. If there was no extra risk of being positive if one was a health-care worker, we would expect the numbers in these two cells to be about the same, disregarding randomly introduced differences from sampling.

If we want to test for the statistical significance of the outcome in a matched study, we use something called McNemar's χ^2 test. If we call the number of pairs in the upper right-hand cell b and the number in the lower left-hand cell c, then the test value becomes:

$$\chi^2 = \frac{(|b - c| - 1)^2}{b + c} \qquad (1 \text{ d.f.})$$

where the straight lines on either side of $|b - c|$ mean that we should take the absolute value of the difference (= disregard the minus sign, if there is one). In our example about hepatitis B, the value would be:

$$\chi^2 = \frac{(|30 - 20| - 1)^2}{30 + 20} = 81 / 50 = 1.62$$

The χ^2 value for McNemar's test has 1 degree of freedom, which means that it has to be greater than 3.84 for our finding to be significant at the 5% level. We conclude that in this matched study, the slight difference in seroprevalence between the groups could easily just be a chance finding.

Just like in the cautionary note about adjusting in the previous section, one should observe that matching only takes care of these potential additional factors that were the basis for the matching. There may well be other confounders involved that we either are not aware of or cannot match for, and these could still distort the result of a study. In fact, one disadvantage with matched studies is that it becomes difficult to control for other confounders in the analysis.

Generally, the introduction of matching in a study requires more work, since many of the potential controls will have to be discarded due to lack of a matching case. In many situations, it becomes simpler to control for confounders in the statistical analysis than to do extensive work trying to find matching controls.

Regression models

Nowadays, most epidemiological studies are analysed with some kind of regression model. A number of computer programmes exist for this purpose with varying degrees of sophistication, including the very powerful packages SAS and GLIM, which require a good deal of knowledge in computing and statistics, and the more immediately accessible EGRET, EpiInfo and JMP (for Macintosh computers).

Regression models are often called 'linear models', or 'multiple regression models'. For the calculation of ORs and RRs one often uses a variant called 'logistic regression models'.

The basic idea in all regression is to fit a line to a number of data points in a diagram. In Fig. 8.1 we assume that we have tested for antibody to some disease in 110 children, 10 from each year group.

% seropositive

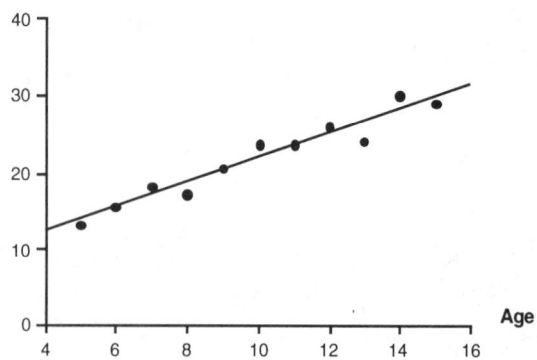

Fig. 8.1 An example of a regression line fitted to a number of data points.

The degree to which such a line fits the data is in principle measured by considering the vertical distances of the points from the line: if all points are quite close to the line this is regarded as a good fit, whereas large distances indicate that the regression line does not describe the data very well.

In epidemiology, the question is usually about effects of exposure. In the example above, we would ask: is there any statistical indication that seropositivity increases with age, or did we get the curve just by chance? If there really was no increase with age, we would assume that the best estimate of seroprevalence in this group would be the overall average, which in this case can be calculated to be 21% for all 110 children. This would also be the expected figure for each age class, and in this case the curve would be as shown in Fig. 8.2.

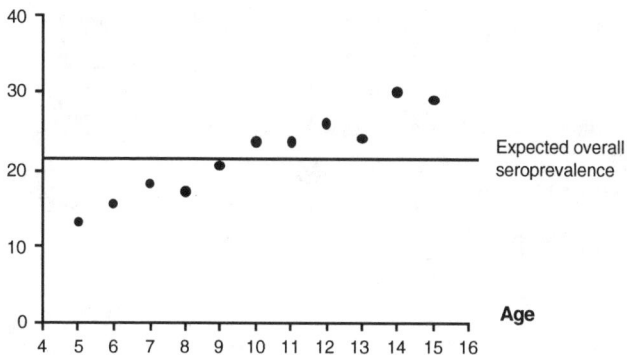

Fig. 8.2 *Same data points as in Fig. 8.1, now with a line showing expected seroprevalence if there were no association between age and seropositivity.*

The statistical analysis then consists of comparing how this last *model*, in which seroprevalence is assumed not to vary with age, fits the data, compared with the model with the sloping line above. The strength of the evidence for the slope model depends partly on the steepness of the slope, partly on the amount of variation around the average value of each year group. In this little example, it seems rather obvious that there is an increase with age.

Even a simple 2×2 table could be analysed like this, but then we would no longer have numerical values along the horizontal axis. Instead there will be two *categories*, as in this example measuring the protective effect of a hypothetical vaccine in a case-control study:

	Vaccinated	**Unvaccinated**	
Ill	20	75	95
Healthy	80	25	105
	100	100	200

The odds of disease will be 20/80 = 0.25 in the vaccinated group, versus 75/25 = 3 in the unvaccinated group. The OR for disease in the unvaccinated would be 3/0.25 = 12, and its statistical significance could be tested by calculating the confidence interval as described in Chapter 4.

A similar calculation could be performed with a regression model. The advantage of this method will not be immediately evident from this simple example, but will be explained below. For reasons of calculation, one often converts the odds into their logarithms when using a regression method, which explains the name 'logistic regression'. The natural logarithms of the odds above are

$$\ln(0.25) = -1.39$$
$$\ln(3) = 1.10$$

and these two values are illustrated as shown in Fig. 8.3.

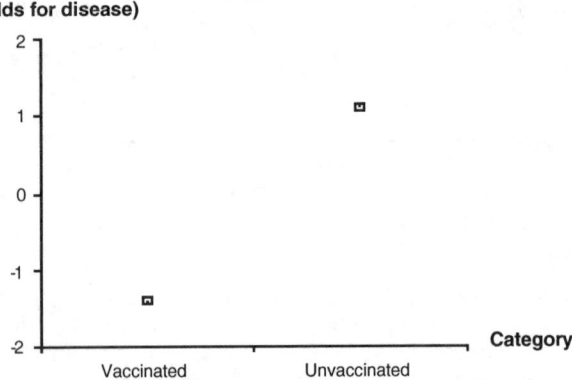

Fig. 8.3 Odds for disease in vaccinated and unvaccinated (logarithms). Does a regression line through the two points fit the data significantly better than a horizontal line through 1n(odds) = − 0.11?

The overall odds for disease among all 200 subjects was 95/105 = 0.90, with the corresponding logarithm $\ln(0.90) = -0.11$. If there was no effect of vaccination on the risk of disease, the expected ln(odds) for both categories would have been − 0.11.

We could now imagine drawing a regression line through the two points above, and comparing it with a horizontal line through ln(odds) = − 0.11. A logistic regression programme will give an estimate for the slope and also a statistical significance value, i.e. the probability that the observed slope just would occur by chance even if the true slope was in reality zero (= the horizontal line). If the vaccinated category is given the value $x = 0$ and the unvaccinated $x = 1$, then the slope would be $(1.10 - [-1.39])/1 = 2.49$. Since subtracting two logarithms amounts to the same thing as taking the logarithm of the quotient, or

$$\ln(a) - \ln(b) = \ln(a/b)$$

this must mean that 2.49 is the logarithm of the two odds divided. But the quotient of the two odds is the definition of the odds ratio, and thus:

$$1.10 - (-1.39) = \ln (3/0.25) = 2.49 = \ln(OR).$$

If $\ln(OR) = 2.49$, exponentiation of both sides gives:

$$e^{\ln(OR)} = OR = e^{2.49} = 12$$

which is the same as the odds ratio calculated from the table.

This may seem a very roundabout way of doing a simple calculation. The strength of regression methods comes from the fact that they directly control for confounders. If we wanted to study the effect of a vaccine as above, we may have to take into account other differences between the two categories in the table. There may be different age distributions in the two groups, for example, the unvaccinated being younger. There may be social differences, for example the unvaccinated coming from poorer backgrounds with larger families, which would mean that they were possibly more exposed, and so on. Let us say that we could divide the children into those younger or older than one year, and into three social classes. In order to control for confounding with nonregression methods we would then have to construct six 2×2 tables like the one above, one for each possible combination of age and social class, thus making a stratified analysis as shown on page 90.

We could then calculate an overall odds ratio for disease in unvaccinated versus vaccinated according to the Mantel–Haenszel procedure described above. This is clearly quite a laborious task, and there might also be some combinations of age and social class for which there were very few subjects in the table, making estimates unreliable.

Age less than one year

Social class 1

	Vaccinated	Unvaccinated
Ill	X	X
Healthy	X	X

Social class 2

	Vaccinated	Unvaccinated
Ill	X	X
Healthy	X	X

Social class 3

	Vaccinated	Unvaccinated
Ill	X	X
Healthy	X	X

Age greater than one year

Social class 1

	Vaccinated	Unvaccinated
Ill	X	X
Healthy	X	X

Social class 2

	Vaccinated	Unvaccinated
Ill	X	X
Healthy	X	X

Social class 3

	Vaccinated	Unvaccinated
Ill	X	X
Healthy	X	X

All this work becomes unnecessary when using a computer programme for logistic regression. One just enters all the subjects, with
vaccination status, age, social class and outcome. The programme
then fits the best possible linear combination to the data, and the OR
for vaccination status given by the programme will be adjusted for
the two other variables.

(For the mathematically inclined, it might be pointed out that the
programme fits a hyperplane in n space through all the data points,
where $n - 1$ is the number of input variables, and the last axis is the
outcome variable. This is most easily visualized for a study with
two variables, say vaccination status along the x axis, age along the
y axis, and outcome along the z axis. Each subject will be a point in

this space, and the algorithm will fit the best plane through all these points. The intersection of this plane with the x-z-plane will be the regression line for outcome versus vaccination status, controlled for age, and the intersection with the y-z-plane will show outcome for different ages, controlled for vaccination status: a regression programme does not differentiate between the variables under study and the confounders, it regards all variables as equal. Incidentally, if you read articles in which regression has been used in the analysis, you may come across the term *covariate*. This word is a favourite with statisticians, and means the same as 'variable' or 'factor', i.e. any of the exposures entered into the regression model to be tested against the outcome. In this parentheses, vaccination status and age would be the two covariates analysed.)

Regression programmes are thus very powerful and efficient. There is, however, one great danger of entering all the data into such a programme, and pressing the 'go' button: the algorithm is essentially a 'black box', and as soon as more than a few variables are included for each subject, it becomes impossible to perceive how the fitting is actually done. It is thus always good epidemiological practice to start the analysis of data with some simple graphs, and some 2×2 tables using rough divisions of the variables, just to get some feel for the data. It is also good practice to let the regression programme analyse the variables under study and the confounders one at a time before they are entered jointly in the model. This strategy is called 'univariate analysis', and usually reveals the most important associations and the strongest confounders. Any major change between an OR or an RR for an exposure given in the univariate analysis and the corresponding adjusted OR or RR should always be investigated. It could be due to strong confounding from another variable, but also to some erroneous assumptions in the model. One such additional problem is called *interaction* and will be the subject of the next section.

Interaction

It is not easy to immediately grasp the assumptions that are usually made when the risk of disease is analysed for several variables simultaneously, either by stratified analysis or by regression models.

One such standard assumption is that risks are added in a multiplicative fashion: suppose that our study shows that persons with risk factor A have twice the risk for disease (adjusted for confounders) than those who do not have risk factor A. We have also found that persons with risk factor B have three times higher risk than those without (still adjusted for confounders). Stratified analysis as well as regression models then postulate that a person who has both A *and* B as risk factors will have 2 × 3 = 6 times higher risk of disease than a person who has neither. Whereas this may be true for a number of exposures and diseases, one really needs knowledge about the actual mechanisms to be able to judge if this assumption is correct. For example, studies have shown that alcoholism and lack of raise in white blood cell count on arrival to hospital both are risk factors for dying from an acute pneumococcal pneumonia. It is not self-evident that a patient with both these risk factors would have the multiplied risk of dying, since one feels that the way in which the factors interplay should be important. Nevertheless, multiplicative risk is implicitly assumed in most epidemiological analyses.

Another standard assumption is that there does exist a true OR or RR for disease from a certain exposure, and that this is independent of the actual values of other variables. This true value might be distorted by confounders but if those are adjusted for properly we should attain a single, dependable value. In a stratified analysis like the one for vaccine efficacy with the six 2 × 2 tables above, the OR for disease according to vaccination status should be the same in each of the six tables. There may be statistical variations between the ORs of the different tables due to sampling, but this is being handled by the Mantel–Haenszel analysis, which gives the best estimate of an overall value from all six tables.

However, there may well be situations when the actual value for an OR or an RR varies with different values for other variables. An example of such *interaction* comes from a study in Brazil, where risk factors for children dying from an infection were analysed in a case-control study.[1] The main objective was to investigate if breastfeeding protected against infant deaths from infectious diseases.

During 1985, data were collected on all infant (less than one year) deaths from infectious causes in an area in southern Brazil. For each case, two infants in the immediate neighbourhood were chosen as controls. The mothers were interviewed about feeding practices, and also about a large number of possible confounders, such as, birth order, birth weight, income, water source, antenatal care, mode of delivery, etc. Adjusted ORs for dying from an infection for those children who were only given milk other than mother's milk were compared with those who were exclusively breast fed (Table 8.3).

Table 8.3 *Odds ratios (ORs) for dying from infectious causes in nonbreast-fed compared to breast-fed children in a study from Brazil.* Source: *Victoria* et al.[1]

	OR	
Diarrhoea	14.2	
Respiratory infection	3.6	
Other infection	2.5	

If however, the ORs were calculated separately for infants aged less than two months and infants aged two to 11 months, the results change (Table 8.4).

Table 8.4 *The same odds ratios as in Table 8.3, now broken down by age group.*

	< 2 months	**2–11 months**
Diarrhoea	23.3	5.3
Respiratory infection	4.1	3.4
Other infection	1.9	2.0

For respiratory and other infections, the influence of feeding practices on the risk of death does not seem to differ much with age. For diarrhoeal deaths, however, there is a huge difference in the evident protection given by breast feeding.

It is interesting to speculate about this difference in risks, and whether the protection is due to anti-infective properties of breast milk, or perhaps to the fact that a breast-fed infant will not come into contact with sources of water that may be contaminated. Which of these mechanisms would most likely explain the difference in risk with age? We will evade those questions here, instead concentrating on the methodological implications of the finding.

How should one give an overall OR for the association between the factor 'not breast feeding' and death from diarrhoea in this study? The answer is that it should probably not be done. The OR for this factor assumes different values in the two different age groups, and to give one value would be misleading, in that it would hide an important interaction between this risk factor and age. Table 8.4 above is telling us something about our study subjects, and this information should not be discarded by just giving an overall OR.

Another example of interaction comes from the study of risk factors for chlamydia infection mentioned in Chapter 7.[2] Some 6,000 young women where interviewed about their sexual lifestyle and tested for asymptomatic chlamydia infection. One question was: 'Have you had any sexually transmitted disease before?' In a univariate analysis, i.e. just comparing prevalence in those who had not previously had any STD to prevalence in those who had, it was found that previous infection was associated with a slightly lower risk of being chlamydia positive in the study (OR = 0.77). When the answers to this question were stratified according to age of the women, the following table of odds for being chlamydia infected in the three age groups emerged.

Table 8.5 *Interaction between the risk factor 'previous sexually transmitted disease (STD)' and age in a study on chlamydia infection in Sweden.* Source: *Ramstedt* et al.[2]

Age group	Previous STD	No previous STD	OR
≤ 17	3.95	1.00	3.95/1.00 = 3.95
18 – 23	1.95	2.74	1.95/2.74 = 0.71
≥ 24	1.44	1.95	1.44/1.95 = 0.74

The table shows that in this group of women, reported previous STD was a strong risk factor for present chlamydia infection among the youngest, whereas in the two older groups there almost seemed to be a protective effect from previous STDs. In this example, the interaction is even more evident than in the example about diarrhoea, since it tends to work in opposite directions in the different strata.

These are two real-life examples of interaction between two variables in an analysis, where the OR for one is not independent of the value for the other. When making a stratified analysis, like the one above, one should always check to see if the ORs for the various strata seem to be very different, which could indicate interaction. In no analysis will the ORs be exactly the same for all strata (look for example on herpes infection in pregnant women in Table 8.1) and the problem is to decide if the variation in ORs is a mere statistical fluctuation around one true value or if there is evidence of interaction. Statistical tests for this problem do exist, but they are not very powerful, and the decision largely remains one of common sense.

In computer programmes for linear regression, there usually exists a possibility to enter interaction variables in the analysis. This is done by indicating which two variables should interact, and then running the model again to see if this improved the regression fit significantly compared with a model with no interaction. Some of the more advanced programmes have built-in algorithms that decide when interaction occurs, but even those do not totally alleviate the necessity for common sense and experience in judging if the assumed interaction is justified by the increase in fit.

Another word for interaction that is sometimes used in epidemiological literature is *effect modification*, which neatly summarizes the concept of the effect of some exposure being modified by the value of another variable.

One practical problem when interaction appears in a study is that the concept may be quite difficult to explain to people with little experience in epidemiology. Tables will become more messy, and it may not be possible to answer straightforward questions about the magnitude of a certain risk.

Misclassification

There is one additional risk with logistic regression models, and that concerns the precision with which we are able to measure the variables analysed. If data on one real risk factor can only be assessed rather crudely, with a high degree of misclassification of individuals, whereas data on a confounder can be measured very precisely, then the regression may show a significant independent influence of risk of disease from the confounder.[3] An example comes from studies of cervical cancer, where one risk factor analysed has been previous STDs and another smoking. If probability of previous STD is assessed as 'number of past sexual partners', this becomes a very crude measure, since the real risk was whether or not any of those were infectious with an STD. Many women will be misclassified by this measure. Smoking, on the other hand, can be assessed rather precisely. The result of such an analysis could be (and has been) that after controlling for number of partners, smoking still remains an independent risk factor. Whereas this may be a true association, it could also be explained by our inability to measure risk of previous STD correctly.

Summary

In many situations one wants to analyse the association between several different factors and risk for disease: age, sex, vaccination status, family size, etc. Epidemiological studies will often collect data on a number of potential risk factors, and the analysis should include the ones thought to be either causally related to the disease or confounders.

Confounding can be controlled by stratification, where the two groups one wants to compare are divided into subgroups, each subgroup consisting of just the subjects who have similar values for the confounder. Comparison is then made, not by comparing the two original big groups, but only the pairs of subgroups with similar values for the confounder. From each pair-wise comparison one gets a value for an OR or an RR, and these values can then be averaged by the Mantel–Haenszel algorithm to give an adjusted value, applicable to the original group comparison.

Matching is another way of controlling for confounding, already from the beginning choosing a control for each case that has similar values for the confounder. The analysis of matched studies becomes a little different.

Most reasonably big data sets are now analysed by some kind of regression method. Their advantage is that they can control for several different confounders simultaneously, and also reveal several independent risk factors. Their main drawback is that the analysis becomes opaque, and that one looses the feel for what is really happening with the data.

If the association between a risk factor and an outcome is influenced by the value of some other risk factor, these two risk factors are said to interact.

References

1. Victora CG, Vaughan JP, Lombardi C, *et al*. Evidence for protection by breast-feeding against infant deaths from infectious diseases in Brazil. *Lancet* 1987; **2**: 319–22.

2. Ramstedt K, Forssman L, Giesecke J, Granath F. Risk factors for *Chlamydia trachomatis* infection in 6810 young women attending family planning clinics. *Int J STD AIDS* 1992; **3**: 117–22.

3. Phillips AN, Davey Smith G. How independent are "independent" effects? Relative risk estimation when correlated exposures are measured imprecisely. *J Clin Epidemiol* 1991; **44**: 1223–31.

9 Survival analysis

Which deals with the study of time periods until something happens, like incubation times, recovery times, etc. An example of how to perform a survival analysis is presented, and the difference between risks and rates is elaborated on.

Often in epidemiology, we are only interested in whether or not something happened, but not exactly when: for example we may want to know *if* someone was infected or not in order to be able to calculate an attack rate, or we may want to know *if* a patient with gastroenteritis ate a specific food item or not in order to calculate an odds ratio. In both these examples it does not matter very much exactly when these events took place. However, in infectious disease epidemiology we are also quite often interested in *when* something occurred. Examples of such questions are calculation of incubation times, or the proportion of a population infected at a given date during an epidemic. We will look more closely at these issues later in this book, but this section introduces the theoretical background to such analyses.

Survival analysis

When one wants to study time periods until something happens, one always starts with a cohort of people that are followed over time, much like in the example of rates and person-years in Chapter 5. We may, for example, want to study the time to death in people who develop cirrhosis from chronic active hepatitis (and this is an example of the type of study that has given this method its name: how many people survive one, two, three, etc. years after developing cirrhosis?). Another recent example that has received much attention is the time from infection with HIV to the development of AIDS, and examples of such studies are given in Chapter 19.

If the durations we are trying to measure are short, like the average incubation time in an outbreak of food poisoning, there is really no need to get into survival analysis. However, if the time periods we are looking at are long or very long, there may be at least three problems with such studies:

1. The outcome we are looking for may not have happened to all people in the cohort. Cohort studies are often lengthy and expensive affairs, and it may not be feasible to continue the project until everyone has developed the disease, or died, etc.

2. We may lose contact with some of the subjects of the study before it is finished, not knowing what happened to them. In most practical situations this becomes more of a problem the longer a study runs. These patients are called 'losses to follow-up', and they always create difficulties in cohort studies. In the example of death from cirrhosis above, we cannot just disregard people who were lost to follow-up as if they had never been in the cohort, since one reason for loosing contact with them may be that they have died from cirrhosis. If such patients were selectively deleted from our cohort, we would underestimate risk of death in the cohort. It might also be the other way around: that some people felt so healthy that they stopped coming to the clinic for follow-ups. If those patients were discarded we would overestimate the risk of death in the cohort.

   However, if many of the subjects who were losses to follow-up remained in the cohort for a long time and we knew that they had not developed the outcome when we lost contact with them, then this fact should contain some information, and it would seem uneconomical not to somehow make use of it.

3. Some people in the cohort may suddenly not be able to develop the outcome: if we are studying death from cirrhosis, then patients who die from other causes cannot take part in the study any longer. If we are studying incidence of hepatitis B infection in a cohort of injecting drug users and one of the subjects gets vaccinated in another clinic, then he cannot give any more information to our study.

As you can see, all the three points above really only relate to problems of cohort studies that are extended in time, but then again, such studies are becoming more and more common even in infectious disease epidemiology.

Terminology

The term 'survival analysis' comes from the original application of this method to demographic data, as when one wants to calculate average life expectancy in a population. But the outcome we are studying does not have to be death, it could be 'becoming infected', or even something positive like 'recovering from an infection', for example hepatitis B carriers becoming antigen negative. We will call the outcome we are studying the *event*, where the event could be something negative or positive to the patient.

Some subjects in our cohort will experience the event, and we can measure the time from the start of the study until this happens for each one of them. However, this will not happen to the subjects in the three groups described above (or at least, we will never know about it for those who are lost to follow-up). These subjects are *censored*, and that could happen for any of the three reasons listed above:

1. The subject had not experienced the event when the study finished.
2. The subject was lost to follow-up from a specified date.
3. The subject experienced an excluding event on a specified date.

For all subjects, whether they were censored or not, we will at least know the time they spent in the cohort. In most clinical studies, the times will be counted as scheduled visits, and if the event is not directly observable by the patient (e.g. loosing HBsAg), it will usually be assumed to have happened on the date of the first visit it was recorded. If the time between visits is long, one sometimes sets the midpoint between the last visit when the event was not observed and the first visit at which it was to be the time of the event. In similar fashion, losses to follow-up should be included only up to the last visit they attended, not to the first one they missed.

An illustrative example

Assume that we want to answer the following question: how long does an injection of gamma globulin protect from infection with hepatitis A in an endemic area?

The simplest way to answer the question would be to give gamma globulin to a large group of people who had not had hepatitis A, send them away to a country where the virus was common, keep them under observation there for a long period, and then record when the cases started to appear. This would be a regular cohort study.

In reality, this would be difficult to achieve, even if studies like these have actually been performed on Western military personnel stationed in tropical countries. A more everyday situation would be that people came to the study country at different times, and stayed there for differing lengths of time. Suppose we chose to study 12 subjects (which is of course far too small a number to achieve any statistical significance, but it will serve for this example) that we knew would be travelling to the endemic country during a 15-month period. They were given gamma globulin just before they left home. Table 9.1 shows what the collected data could look like.

Table 9.1 *Example of input data for a survival analysis. Twelve subjects were given gamma globulin just before they departed to a hepatitis A endemic area, and were subsequently followed for varying lengths of time*

Subject	Departed month	Diagnosed month	Comment
1	2	11	-
2	9	-	Still abroad, healthy
3	3	-	Returned home in month 8, healthy
4	1	-	Lost contact in month 3
5	1	-	Still abroad, healthy
6	10	-	Returned home in month 13, healthy
7	6	-	Received new dose of gamma in month 7
8	4	8	-
9	3	-	Returned home in month 4, healthy
10	8	-	Lost contact in month 13
11	7	13	-
12	13	-	Still abroad, healthy

Figure 9.1 displays this data in a graph, with time along the x axis and each person as a line, just as we did in Chapter 5 (see Fig. 5.1). The infections (= events) are marked by a short vertical line at the end of the corresponding line.

Subjects 1, 8 and 11 experienced the event (i.e. they had hepatitis A), all the others are censored:

• subjects 2, 5 and 12 because they had not experienced the event at the end of the study period,
• subjects 4 and 10 because they were lost to follow-up,
• subjects 3, 6 and 9 because they were not exposed any longer, and
• subject 7 because he received a new dose of gamma globulin, which invalidated the experiment.

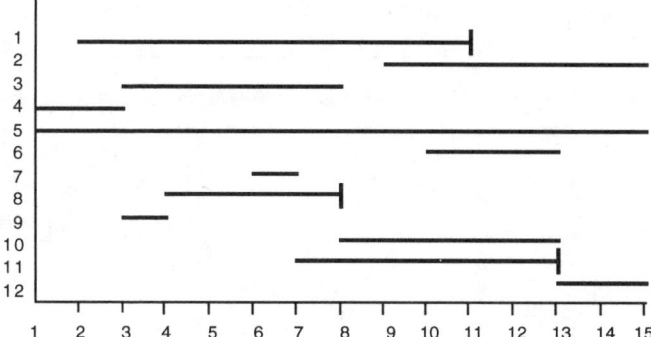

Fig. 9.1 *Line diagram representing 12 people given gamma globulin. A short, vertical bar indicates an event, in this case the diagnosis of a hepatitis A infection.*

The graph looks rather messy. One obvious thing to do, since we are not interested in exact dates but rather time in the cohort, would be to imagine that everyone had the same time of entry, namely the day they were injected. This would correspond to pulling all the lines in the graph to the left border. At the same time, we rearrange the order of the subjects according to length of stay(see Fig. 9.2).

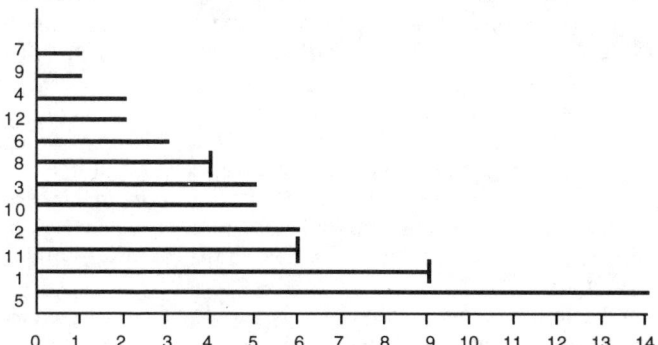

Fig. 9.2 *The same group of people as in Fig. 9.1, but this time ordered after length of follow-up in the study.*

We see that no case appears before four months of stay, but that after that time, people start getting hepatitis A infections. One person stays for 14 months without becoming infected.

We could rearrange Table 9.1 in the same way, letting 'I' stand for infected, and 'C' for censored, where we no longer differentiate between the reasons for censoring (Table 9.2).

Table 9.2 *Same subjects as in Table 9.1, now arranged according to follow-up time. 'C' denotes censored, 'I' infected*

Subject	Months in study	Outcome
7	1	C
9	1	C
4	2	C
12	2	C
6	3	C
8	4	I
3	5	C
10	5	C
2	6	C
11	6	I
1	9	I
5	14	C

The survival curve we want to construct is the chance of still being uninfected after a certain number of months in the cohort. (Or conversely, the risk of having become infected after a number of months.)

The way to calculate that is to make a new table, Table 9.3, as follows:

1. List all the months according to the above table, using months in the cohort for each subject, not the actual calendar month of the happenings.
2. In the second column, list how many people were left in the cohort at the beginning of that month. Call that number N_i, where N_1 is the number in the first row, N_2 in the second, and so on.
3. In the third column, list how many events (infections in this case) happened during that month. Call that number I_i, where I_1 is the first row, I_2 the second, etc. For several of the months, I_i will just be a zero.
4. In the fourth column list how many people (if any) were censored during that month.

In our example, the table thus far would look like Table 9.3. This table should read: in the first line, we see that 12 people entered the cohort. Two of these were censored during the first month. The second line thus shows that 10 people remained in the cohort at the beginning of the second month, and that two of these were censored during that month. The first event appeared in month 4, line 4. You can see that each N_i is equal to the N_i in the line above minus the events and censorings in that line.

Table 9.3 *The first steps in the construction of a table for the survival analysis in Table 9.1. 'N$_i$' denotes the number of subjects still under observation at the beginnig of each month, 'I$_i$' the number of events and 'Censored' the number of censorings during that month*

Month	N_i	I_i	Censored
1	12	0	2
2	10	0	2
3	8	0	1
4	7	1	0
5	6	0	2
6	4	1	1
7	2	0	0
8	2	0	0
9	2	1	0
10	1	0	0
11	1	0	0
12	1	0	0
13	1	0	0
14	1	0	1

At the beginning of each month there is obviously a number, N_i, who could fall ill during that month. In some of the months one of the subjects is diagnosed with hepatitis infection, in some not. The best estimate of the risk of becoming a case during month *i* is the number of cases during that month divided by the number of subjects at its beginning, or I_i/N_i. The probability of *not* becoming a case during month *i* is obviously the converse: $N_i - I_i$ subjects out of the total N_i did not become infected, and the 'risk of not becoming infected' will thus be $(N_i - I_i)/N_i = 1 - I_i/N_i$. Any subject who was still healthy at the beginning of month *i* would have the chance $(1 - I_i/N_i)$ of remaining healthy at the end of the month.

A basic fact of statistical theory is that the collective chance of A and B and C happening is the same as the chance that A happens, multiplied by the chance that B happens, multiplied by the chance that C happens. In our example, this would mean that the chance of remaining healthy after, say, three time periods can be calculated as the chance of escaping infection during the first period, multiplied by the chance of remaining healthy during the second period, multiplied by the chance of not becoming a case during the third period.

This is all a bit difficult when described in words like this. It becomes simpler when one uses mathematics:

5. Next, in a fifth column, calculate $1 - I_i/N_i$ for each line. Call this number L_i (where the 'L' stands for being lucky and escaping disease). For the months when there are no cases, L_i will just be equal to 1.

6. Finally, call the numbers of the sixth column S_i (where 'S' stands for survival). They are calculated by multiplying the S_i in the line above with the L_i to the left (i.e. $S_{i+1} = S_i \times L_{i+1}$). For the first line, S_1 is defined as $L_1 \times 1$. Each S_i is an estimate of the chance of still remaining uninfected just at the end of the corresponding month.

The final table, Table 9.4, becomes:

Table 9.4 *The final table for the survival analysis in Table 9.1. S_i is an estimate of the probability of remaining uninfected at the end of each month*

Time point	N_i	I_i	Censored	$1 - I_i/N_i$	S_i
1	12	0	2	1	1
2	10	0	2	1	1
3	8	0	1	1	1
4	7	1	0	0.86	0.86
5	6	0	2	1	0.86
6	4	1	1	0.75	0.64
7	2	0	0	1	0.64
8	2	0	0	1	0.64
9	2	1	0	0.5	0.32
10	1	0	0	1	0.32
11	1	0	0	1	0.32
12	1	0	0	1	0.32
13	1	0	0	1	0.32
14	1	0	1	1	0.32

Figure 9.3 shows how the S_i:s are plotted against time to get the survival curve (often called the Kaplan–Meier plot, after its inventors).

This curve quite nicely sums up what we want to know: it shows that infections start appearing some four months after the injection with gamma globulin, and that the risk of becoming a case increases rather linearly after that. The median time till being diagnosed seems to be some nine months. (The risk of becoming infected with hepatitis A in this hypothetical country must be very high, and the gamma globulin seems to wear off more quickly than in real life, so please do not take this as a very realistic example.)

% still healthy

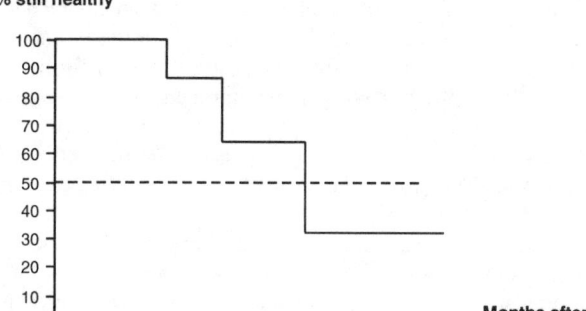

Fig. 9.3 *A Kaplan–Meier plot showing the survival curve for the data in Table 9.1.*

The further to the right we move along the survival curve, the less subjects will be left on which to base our estimates of L_i and S_i. This means that the latter part of such a curve will always be more uncertain than the first part. It is good practice to indicate the number of subjects still at risk after each event on the curve to give the reader some feeling for the statistical uncertainty of the plotted curve (this has e.g. been done for the survival curves in Chapter 19).

Survival curves can be compared by statistical tests to see if, for example, the curves are different for one group receiving some kind of treatment versus an untreated group, but we will not go into such tests here.

If you have any familiarity with spread-sheet programmes for a personal computer, you can see that it is really quite easy to perform a survival analysis with such a programme. Times, events and censorings are entered in separate columns, and three simple repeated formulae calculate the N_i, L_i and S_i for each line.

The difference between risk and rate

Another way to analyse the data in the above example would be to calculate the rate of infection per person month, just as we did in the little example in Chapter 5. Let us first look a bit more stringently at the definition of rates.

Rate is really an instantaneous measure, and as such, rather an abstraction. It has been compared to the actual value on the speedometer of a car: even if the needle points at 72 km/hour right now, that does not mean that we will travel exactly 72 km during the next hour – it is just the speed at which we are driving for the moment.

Rate is always calculated as the proportion who fall ill out of those who are susceptible at that precise moment in time, which means that if people are infected and becoming immune, then the number of susceptibles in the denominator is decreasing with time (in epidemiological literature, the number of susceptibles is often called 'number at risk').

An example: let us assume that herpes simplex virus type 1 infects a population of 100 children at a constant rate. Initially, they are all susceptible, and during the first year of our study we diagnose 12 cases. This means that the risk of getting herpes during one year is $12/100 = 0.12$, or 12%, which might seem reasonable. However, if we extrapolate to 10 years it appears as if the risk of getting herpes will be 120%, which cannot be true since a risk can never be higher than 100%.

Just as has been mentioned before, a figure for a risk must always include the time period we are considering. If exposure to a pathogen is continuous, then the probability of observing an infection in a study subject will obviously be greater the longer he/she is followed. In an influenza epidemic lasting from November through February, the risk of becoming infected in November will be less than the risk of becoming infected at any time during the four-month epidemic.

If we instead calculate the rate, this problem of having to state the time period of observation can be evaded: assume that the 12 cases in the herpes example above appear evenly over the year. We will then follow 100 children for one month, but after this one child will have had an infection with herpes type 1. We then follow 99 susceptibles for another month, but after that one more will have had the disease. We thus follow 98 children for the third month, and so on.

The total number of person-months added during the one-year study will thus be: $100 + 99 + 98 + 97 + ... + 90 + 89 = 1134$. This means that the rate is $12/1134 = 0.0106$, or 1.06% per person-month. Just as in the example with speed, it does not matter which time unit we choose to measure rate; a speed of 72 km/hour is the same as 1.2 km/minute, or 20 m/s. A rate of 1.06% per person-month is thus equal to $12 \times 1.06 = 12.7\%$ per person-year. We see that the rate per year is slightly higher than the risk of getting herpes during one year. (Mathematically, this is due to the fact that the denominator for calculation of risk is the original 100 children, whereas the denominator in the rate calculation decreases with the number of children who get herpes infection during the year.)

The way to get from rate to risk is by the following formula:

$$\text{Risk} = 1 - e^{-\text{Rate} \times \text{time}}$$

where time is measured in the same unit as risk and rate. The risk of getting a herpes type 1 infection during 10 years in this example would thus be:

$$\text{Risk in 10 years} = 1 - e^{-0.127 \times 10} = 1 - 0.28 = 0.72$$

or a bit below 100%, which appears reasonable: a few people will always escape infection. (Parenthetically, we can also see that the risk during one year is:

$$1 - e^{-0.127 \times 1} = 1 - 0.88 = 0.12 \text{ or } 12\%$$

just as we calculated at the outset.)

Many diseases are so rare that the difference between risk and rate becomes negligible. If one out of every 100,000 persons in a country get meningococcal meningitis each year, this does not change the number at risk appreciably, and in this case the risk *and* the rate are both 1/100,000 per year.

Now to get back to the hepatitis A example that we have spent the greater part of this chapter analysing by survival methods. The number of person-months in this study is easily calculated from the second table in the example: the total for all the 12 subjects is 58. There were three people infected with hepatitis A virus, and the rate thus becomes 3/58 cases per person-month = 0.05, meaning that there was just below a 5% risk of becoming infected during each month in the high-endemic country. If we multiply this figure by 12 we get 0.62, which is the rate of infection per person-year.

This is also an interesting figure, but it fails to reveal the important fact shown in the Kaplan-Meier graph above, namely that there were no infections at all during the first three to four months. When rates are being calculated as above, it is always assumed that the incidence rate is constant over time. The survival analysis gives much more information about changes in rate over time.

Summary

The distribution of time periods until some positive or negative event occurs is best studied in cohorts of subjects, and analysed with survival analysis. This is especially true if the times are long, and there will be considerable problems with losses to follow-up during the study. In survival analysis, the time in the cohort is divided into smaller units, like months or years, and for each time unit the number of subjects who could experience the event under study (e.g. the number of subjects still in the cohort who are susceptible) are compared to the actual number of events during the time period (e.g. the number of cases). This ratio becomes an estimate of the incidence during this time unit. All time units are then put together to get an overall survival curve, which is often plotted as a Kaplan–Meier graph.

Figures for risks always, implicitly or explicitly, refer to a certain time period. By calculating rates, it becomes possible to get an incidence measure that is independent of time period. However, when rates are calculated as number of events per person-month or person-year, constant incidence rate is assumed, and variations in incidence over time become more evident from a Kaplan–Meier plot.

10 Mathematical models for epidemics

Here we are introduced to the mathematical background to the theory of epidemics. A simple model for an epidemic is presented, and the restrictions of such models are discussed. The importance of contact patterns and immunity for the shape of an epidemic – or endemic – is underlined.

One of the perpetual dreams of mankind has always been to be able to predict the future. The regular recurrence of epidemics, and the similar shapes of consecutive epidemics of a disease have for a long time tempted people with a mathematical inclination to make some kind of model. One need only look at the graph for reported cases of measles in England and Wales before the introduction of vaccine, to see that there is a very clear pattern here (Fig. 10.1).

Cases per quarter

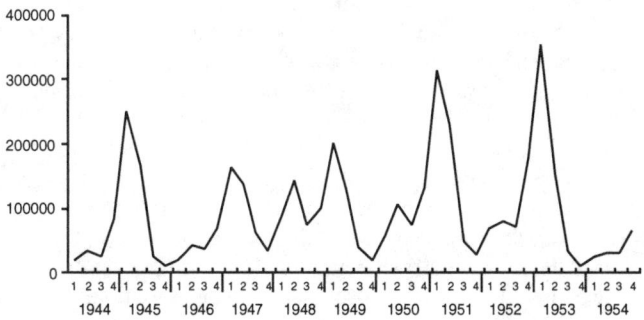

Fig. 10.1 *Quarterly reported cases of measles in England and Wales 1944–1954.*

With the exception of 1948, the epidemic peaks evidently occur every second year, and the highest number of cases during an epidemic always seems to be in the first quarter of the year. The curves for the two periods 1950–51 and 1952–53 are strikingly similar. Surely, there must be some way of describing this pattern in mathematical terms – to make some kind of model of measles incidence, which could then be used to predict future epidemics.

If this way of thinking about infectious diseases in terms of models seems somewhat unfamiliar, one should only consider all the results of similar models that we meet daily in other circumstances:

One of the most complex examples is given by the weather forecasts, which are made using supercomputers, where large systems of equations are linked to huge libraries of previous meteorological patterns. The present situation is compared with these data, and the most probable future course calculated. Another ramification has been to try and predict sociological developments, for although the future actions of an individual may be impossible to foresee, it might be feasible to say something about how large groups of people will behave. This type of model is best represented by the economical forecasts that regularly come out of banks and financial institutions. The fact that these forecasts rarely turn out to agree with the actual economical development does not seem to diminish their news value: a good example of our insatiable need to see into the future.

In contrast to the prophecies of cards or crystal balls, such predictions about the future as are based on a scientific way of thinking are often phrased in mathematical terms. This can make them difficult to understand for the nonmathematician, and it also lends them an air of exactitude that they may not always merit. No model will be better than the assumptions on which it was built, and these assumptions are usually quite easy to understand and question, even if the formulae look deterring. It is sometimes difficult to see the exact assumptions underlying the model, but in any good publication they should be stated clearly.

Models can be useful for other purposes than predictions. By giving a simplified picture of a development, where less important factors have been removed, they can aid us in understanding complex contexts. They may consequently also help us to realize which factors are the most important determinants of the development, and which we thus should study closer and try to measure more exactly.

Finally, models make quite good tools for teaching infectious disease epidemiology.

Basic reproductive rate

We have already come across the concept of reproductive rate in Chapter 2, and we have seen that it measures the potential for an infection to spread in a population.

Figure 10.2 shows a schematic spread of an infectious disease.

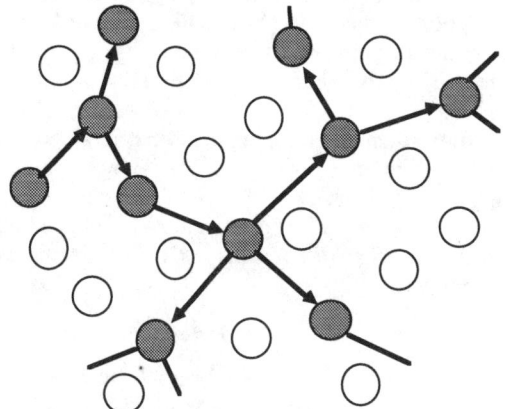

***Fig. 10.2** A schematic spread of an infection in a population.*

The disease is brought into the group by the person at the left border. He infects one person, who in turn infects two others. One of these does not spread the infection, but the other infects one more, and so on. We see that the average number of persons directly infected by each case is:

$$(1 + 2 + 0 + 1 + 3 + 2 + 1 + 1 + 2 + 1 + 2)/10 = 1.5$$

The *basic* reproductive rate is called R_o and has a strict definition:

R_o is the average number of persons directly infected by an infectious case during his entire infectious period, when he enters a totally susceptible population.

The reason for including the clause 'totally susceptible population' in the definition of basic reproductive rate is the following: if the disease is one that confers immunity after infection, then the number of susceptible persons in the population will decrease with time, and more and more of an infectious person's contacts will be with people who are already immune. The actual reproductive rate thus decreases as the infection spreads, but the *basic* rate is unaffected by this.

Obviously, R_0 is rather an abstraction. In order to calculate an average R_0, we would first introduce an infectious case into a population and count the number of secondary cases. We would then have to turn the population back to its original, totally susceptible state, introduce another case, count secondary cases, and so on. The strict definition above thus becomes quite theoretical, but we can usually get a good estimate of R_0 by counting the secondary cases as long as the number of already immune contacts is negligible.

Once an epidemic is under way, the present reproductive rate is usually denoted just by R.

If a new disease enters a population, what is its probability of spreading? From the above reasoning, it may not come as a total surprise that the necessary condition for an epidemic is that R_0 is greater than 1. In words, this means that every infected person on average infects more than one new person. In fact, the three possible situations are these:

$$R_0 < 1 \Rightarrow \text{ the disease will eventually disappear}$$

$$R_0 = 1 \Rightarrow \text{ the disease will become endemic}$$

$$R_0 > 1 \Rightarrow \text{ there will be an epidemic}$$

If $R_0 < 1$, then every new wave of infection in the population will consist of fewer people than the one before, and eventually the disease will die out. If R_0 is equal to 1, then there will be approximately the same number of people infected all the time, which is the definition of an endemic, and if $R_0 > 1$ there will be an ever increasing number of infected people.

Now let us see what happens if people become immune after infection: let us assume that R_0 for a disease is 2, i.e. in the beginning every case infects on average two susceptible individuals. As time goes by more and more people are becoming immune, and at some time point half the population will have become immune to the disease. This means that of all the contacts an infectious case will have with other people, only one half will actually transmit the infection, and R will have fallen from the original value of 2 to 1. As even more people become immune, the actual R will continue to fall below 1, and the epidemic will eventually die out.

This way of reasoning has important implications for the issue of vaccination coverage. If we, instead of letting the natural infection gradually increase the proportion of immune as above, vaccinate the population against a disease, what proportion of the population must be vaccinated in order to prevent an epidemic? Well, if the basic reproduction rate is R_0, this means that on average R_0 contacts will be infected by someone who has the infection. Consider we have a disease for which $R_0 = 4$ in a susceptible population. In the unvaccinated, natural stage, a primary case of disease will thus infect four people. However, if 25% of the population have already been vaccinated against the disease, then one of the four people that *should* have become infected by the primary case will escape infection. (Remember that we are always talking about averages when considering R_0, and on average one out of every four potential secondary cases will be protected by the vaccination.) In this, partly vaccinated, population the index case will thus only infect three people on average.

If half the population has been vaccinated, then the primary case will only infect two people, and if 75% have been vaccinated, there will only be one secondary case, on average. We see that if 75% have been vaccinated, there will be a kind of endemic situation in the early stages, with each infectious case infecting one more, on average. (After the infection has spread for a while, the actual R will of course drop below 1, since more and more are becoming naturally immunized.)

Now comes the crucial bit: if *more* than three quarters of the population have been vaccinated, then right from the beginning there will be less than one new case per infectious individual, on average, and the epidemic can not even begin to spread.

This example was for an R_0 of 4. We could generalize the argument to any R_0: assume that the proportion p of the population have already been vaccinated. Out of the R_0 people that *should* have become infected by this person bringing the disease into the population, $p \times R_0$ will thus escape infection. The number of people that *will* become infected by the primary case is thus, on average, $R_0 - p \times R_0$.

If we want to be certain that the disease will not spread in an epidemic fashion, we want the number of secondary cases from this one infectious primary case to be less than 1, on average. What does this tell us about p, the level of vaccination required?

The number of secondary cases $R_0 - p \times R_0$ should be less than 1:

$$R_0 - p \times R_0 < 1,$$

which is equal to:

$$R_0 - 1 < p \times R_0$$

or:

$$p > \frac{R_0 - 1}{R_0} = 1 - \frac{1}{R_0}$$

We have here shown a fundamental formula for vaccination protection: in order to prevent epidemics of a disease, the proportion of the population that must be vaccinated is higher than 1 minus the inverse of the basic reproductive rate.

It is very important to understand that this vaccination level will not prevent *all* secondary cases of the disease. Unless vaccination coverage is 100%, there will always be some secondary, and even tertiary, cases from newly introduced infectious sources. What we have shown is that with this vaccination level, there cannot be any real epidemics in this population. Any little 'microepidemic' arising round an infectious case will soon die out on its own.

Take measles as an example. In a susceptible Western population, R_0 for this disease has been shown to be around 15, i.e. every case of measles will infect 15 other people, on average. Then the formula predicts that if we want to prevent measles epidemics, more than $1 - 1/15 = 0.94$ or 94% of the population must be vaccinated.

The level of immunity in a population, which prevents epidemics (even if some transmissions may still occur) is called *herd immunity*. The higher R_0 is for a disease, the higher proportion of the population will have to be vaccinated to achieve herd immunity, which seems rather logical.

These calculations could seem somewhat theoretical, but almost exactly this line of reasoning was used when the WHO devised a strategy to eradicate smallpox in the 1960s, or when there was a resolution to eradicate measles from the USA at about the same time.

What determines R_0?

I have repeatedly stressed above that R_0 is always an average value, where the number of transmissions from each infectious person is averaged. This means that if there are large differences in the rate of spread within different subgroups of the population, the average R_0 will be quite useless. The concept of R_0 finds its greatest use for the description of diseases that are spread broadly among people meeting more or less at random.

The basic formula that gives the actual value of R_0 is:

$$R_0 = \beta \times \mathbf{k} \times \mathbf{D}$$

where β is the risk of transmission per contact (i.e. basically the attack rate), **k** is the number of potentially infectious contacts that the average person in the population has per time unit, and **D** is the duration of infectivity of an infected person, measured in the same time unit as **k** was.

We will now dissect this formula, to see what it means: β, the transmission risk per contact, is of course different for different diseases and different types of contacts. Taking HIV infection as an example, we could say that β for the contact 'shaking hands' is zero, the infection is not transmitted that way. For sexual intercourse, β is probably somewhere between 0.001 and 0.1, and for the contact 'blood transfusion', which could be seen as a very close contact between the donor and the recipient, β is virtually = 1.0.

Table 3.3 from Hope Simpson's studies of childhood diseases gave examples of household attack rates for three diseases:

Measles	0.80
Chicken pox	0.72
Mumps	0.38

In this case 'contact' should be taken to mean 'being siblings in the same household', and it is probable that the β's would be lower for more casual contacts.

Many public health measures to prevent the spread of infections aim at decreasing β, such as using a condom, wearing a face mask, or washing one's hands.

k – the average number of contacts a person has per time unit – is of course also different for different diseases. In a measles outbreak in a school, it could be the average number of children any child passes per day. For a sexually transmitted disease, it would be the number of new partners per month or year. In the spread of a common cold, it would be the number of people an infected person sneezes at, or even just shakes hands with during one day.

Isolation of cases is a public health measure which aims at decreasing **k**, even though it may often not be very effective. Public campaigns that recommend people to have fewer sexual partners is another example.

D, the average duration of infectivity, is a biological constant for any disease. With antibiotics, it is often possible to shorten **D**, and this is one of the instances where infectious disease epidemiology is rather special: treatment of ill people actually diminishes the risk to others. It should be noted, though, that this is not true for all infections;

antibiotics for a salmonella infection does not seem to influence the time a person remains a carrier.

The formula above is really quite trivial: the more infectious a disease is, and the more people a case meets, and the longer he is infective, the higher the rate of secondary infections will be. It is, however, often enlightening to dissect an epidemic situation in this formal way.

An example: imagine a sexually transmitted disease, which in a certain population has an R_0 of 1.2, and which would therefore build up to an epidemic. If we could get just one quarter of all couples to use a condom, and assume that β would be $= 0$ in those contacts, R would fall to 0.9 and the disease would eventually disappear.

An approximate formula for R_0

From these discussions it should be clear that the higher the R_0 is for an infection that is spread broadly in society by everyday contacts, the greater the risk will be of meeting this infection early in life. If the transmission risk is high, and if many people are infectious, chances are that many children will be infected. In fact, it is just those infections that have a high R_0 and that confer long immunity that we call childhood diseases, since practically everyone is exposed and infected in childhood, but subsequently protected from disease.

For such diseases there exists a simple approximate formula to estimate R_0 from knowledge of average age at infection:[1]

$$R_0 = 1 + \frac{L}{A}$$

where L is average life span of the individuals in the population, and A is average age at infection. You can see that if average life expectancy at birth is 70 years, a disease for which average age at infection is seven years would have an R_0 of 11. If measles has an R_0 of 15 in Western countries as stated above, then this formula should give average age at infection to be around five years, which seems reasonable.

A simple model

Most of the mathematical models on infectious diseases that have been published concern childhood diseases, i.e. illnesses that are highly contagious, have short incubation periods and short durations, and confer immunity after infection. We will look at such a model here, making the following assumptions:

- the population is fixed, so that no one enters and no one leaves or dies
- the incubation period is zero, and
- the duration of infectivity is just as long as the clinical disease.

The illness is brought into the group by someone who broke the first rule temporarily, and contracted it outside.

We call the size of the population N. At any time, it can be divided into three proportions:

- S, which is the proportion of N that is susceptible
- I, which is the proportion currently infected and infectious
- R, which is the proportion immune (calling this 'R' is an old custom, it stands for 'resistant').

Before the first case is infected, S is obviously $= 1$, since everyone is susceptible, and I and R are both $= 0$. As the epidemic spreads, S will decrease and R will increase. Intuitively, I should first increase, and then decrease.

We will now set up three equations to show how these three proportions will change over time. In doing this, we will use the time derivatives of the proportions. This is written

$$\frac{dX}{dt}, \text{ where } X \text{ could be } S, I \text{ or } R$$

If you are unfamiliar with this notation, just read it as 'the rate at which X is presently changing'. If there is a minus sign in front of the derivative, this means that X is presently decreasing, otherwise it is increasing.

At any time during the epidemic, the three equations will be:

$$\frac{dS}{dt} = -\beta \times \mathbf{k} \times S \times I \tag{1}$$

$$\frac{dI}{dt} = -\beta \times \mathbf{k} \times S \times I - \frac{I}{\mathbf{D}} \tag{2}$$

$$\frac{dR}{dt} = \frac{I}{\mathbf{D}} \tag{3}$$

Let us look at these equations, one at a time. The first one says that the number of susceptibles is decreasing (minus sign), just as we guessed. However, the actual rate of decrease, $\beta \times \mathbf{k} \times S \times I$, deserves an explanation. Look at the $S \times I$ part first. In the population, there are six different types of contacts possible:

- susceptible meets susceptible
- susceptible meets infectious
- susceptible meets resistant (immune)
- infectious meets infectious
- infectious meets resistant, and
- resistant meets resistant.

Obviously, transmission can only occur in the second type (susceptible meets infectious). If all contacts take place completely at random, the proportion of all contacts that occur between members of two groups will be the product of these two groups' respective proportions, i.e. $S \times I$ in this case. To give an example: if 30% of the population belong to the susceptible group, there will be at least one susceptible involved in 30% of all contacts. If another 10% are infectious, they will make up 10% of all the contacts that the susceptible group has, and thus 0.30 x 0.10 = 0.03 or 3% of *all* contacts in the total group will be between susceptible and infectious. (Similarly, 0.30 x 0.30 = 0.09 or 9% of all contacts will be between two susceptibles, and 1% between two infectious.)

$\mathbf{k}$ is the average number of contacts any person in the population has, say per day. Out of all these contacts, just the fraction $S \times I$ will be of the type that could result in a transmission, and $\mathbf{k} \times S \times I$ is thus the number of potentially infectious contacts per day. Finally, to get the number of transmission actually occurring, we multiply by β which is the risk of transmission in each of these contacts.

In the second equation, the first term on the right-hand side says that the number of infecteds increases at the same rate as the susceptibles become infected, which is obvious. However, after the time $\mathbf{D}$, an infected person turns immune, and is taken out of the infectious group, so that if $\mathbf{D}$ equals 10 days, then 1/10 of all the infecteds become immune each day.

The third equation just says that exactly the same number of people that leave the infectious group because they become immune are entering the resistant group.

Let us see how these equations appear graphically. Assume that the disease has a transmission probability of 0.15 ($=\beta$), that people in this population have on average 12 contacts per week ($= \mathbf{k}$), and that the disease lasts 1 week ($=\mathbf{D}$). As before, the incubation period is zero, and the period of infectivity is just as long as the disease span. We start with 1,000 people, and introduce one infectious case on week 1. The number of susceptibles can then be read from the graph (Fig. 10.3).

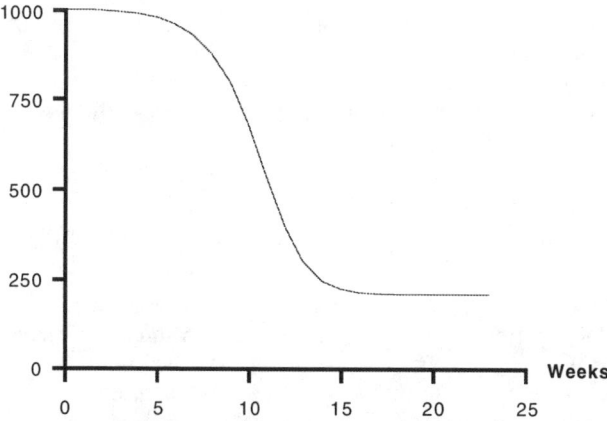

Fig. 10.3 *Weekly number of susceptibles in an imaginary epidemic in a closed population of 1,000 people. The epidemic starts with one infectious person being introduced at time zero.*

The epidemic starts off slowly, since there are few infectious cases around. Around week 11, it reaches its maximum incidence rate of some 140 new cases per week, but then it slows down again, this time due to lack of susceptibles. By week 16 or 17, the epidemic has subsided. Note that some 200 individuals will escape the infection.

The entire course of the epidemic for all three groups is illustrated in Fig. 10.4.

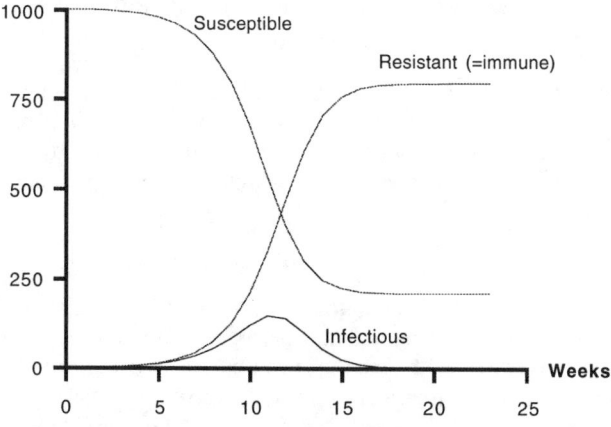

Fig. 10.4 *Same imaginary epidemic as in Fig. 10.3, but now also including weekly numbers of infectious and immune.*

The curve for the number of resistant persons is rather the inverse of the susceptible curve, which makes sense. At the end there will be some 800 people who have become immune. The proportion of the population that is infectious at any one time never exceeds 15%.

Using the basic formula above $R_0 = \beta \times \mathbf{k} \times \mathbf{D}$, we would get for this epidemic

$$R_0 = 0.15 \times 12 \times 1 = 1.8$$

which shows that even this rather low R_0 can give rise to a substantial epidemic. What happens is that somewhere around week 11, the actual R falls below 1, and at that point the epidemic starts to tail off.

The fact that not everyone will contract the infection seems counterintuitive: how could 200 people of the 1,000 in the above example escape infection when as many as 140 subjects may be infectious at any one time? This lack of total incidence was already noted in smallpox outbreaks in the last century, and one theory that received a lot of support well into this century was that the pathogen grew progressively less virulent after repeated passages through individuals. A virus or bacteria would thus be more virulent (higher β) when passing from the primary to a secondary case than when passing from generation 10 to generation 11, and this would explain why the outbreak subsided before everyone was hit. However, the line of reasoning behind the above very simple model makes it clear that this assumption of decreasing virulence is really not necessary. Seen from the point of view of the epidemic, every infectious subject will be given a certain number of potentially infective exposures to use on other people. As the number of immune increases, more and more of these exposures will be 'thrown away' on nonsusceptibles, and even if an exposure is used on a susceptible there is just the probability β that a transmission will actually occur. In some sense, the remaining susceptibles will be protected by the large number of immune around them, which is the concept of herd immunity introduced above.

Objections to the model

At least two of the basic assumptions underlying this model are seriously unrealistic. The first is that every person in the population will meet every other with equal probability. This may be true for atoms in a mixture of gases, and the formulation of the model above actually derives from chemistry, where the 'law of mass action' describes how substances enter into chemical reactions.

Among people there will always be some contacts that are likely or common, and others that will never occur. One's family is such a 'subgroup' for infectious disease spread, and if you remember the monkey pox example in Chapter 3, the researchers calculated different attack rates for family contacts and more distant contacts. Other important subgroups are the school, the workplace, one's friends, etc. Differences in age and geographical distances will have major influences on who meets whom. The fact that the contact pattern in society is far from homogeneous will result in most infections spreading more slowly than the model above predicts. Furthermore, it is quite conceivable that contact patterns change once one becomes ill: one only has to go to bed for a couple of days with the infection to decrease the number of contacts substantially.

Another problem is that the epidemic itself may well influence the contact pattern. The most difficult thing to model concerning HIV spread is to what degree the public's changing habits in face of the epidemic will themselves lead to the epidemic taking another course.

The second unrealistic assumption is that only one kind of contact exists, with a given β. As discussed briefly above, diseases may spread along different routes with varying degrees of transmission risk. If subgroups of the population have very different contact modes, there can be very different outcomes of an introduction of a disease into these groups. For HIV, anal intercourse and blood-to-blood contact through the sharing of needles carry a higher β than vaginal intercourse. This implies that in a group of homosexual men, or of intravenous drug users, there may be a higher risk of epidemic spread than in a nondrug-using heterosexual subgroup of the population, even at the same contact rate.

Again, this takes us back to the sociology of infectious diseases. The potential for an epidemic lies not only with the biological constants of the disease, such as transmission risk or duration, but just as much with the way society is organized: how we travel, the size of our families, the division of the school year, the density of the population, etc. Many of the epidemics that in the past were perceived as 'new' diseases probably owed their emergence to changing contact patterns (faster intercontinental travel, increasing population density, etc.). Since mankind has been mixing with its bacteria and viruses for at least a couple of hundred thousand years, the probability of new pathogens suddenly emerging should be rather low. However, it seems to be a historical fact that we fail to see how *we* change, and how that gives ground for disease spread.

This is with all probability true also for the future: there are right now pathogens out there leading their quiet lives, who are only waiting for us humans to change our ways of life so that they will find an ecological niche in our society.

The role of chance

The way of thinking about infectious diseases used above is *deterministic*. This means that the development and size of an epidemic are always determined by β, $\mathbf{k}$, and $\mathbf{D}$. Every time our model disease in the graphs above is introduced into a susceptible population, the ensuing epidemic will run the same course.

For established epidemics in large populations a deterministic model may not be too wrong, but it is intuitively clear that chance may play a major role, especially early in an epidemic. If someone with measles comes to an island where only a few are immune, he would start an epidemic according to the deterministic model. If, however, he only happens to meet immune persons before he recovers, there will be no epidemic at all.

Models that take account of chance are called *probabilistic*, and often become more mathematically complex than deterministic models. They are often evaluated using a computer, where a simulated epidemic is run many times. Each run creates a different result due to chance, and these results can be averaged to find the most likely course.

For both deterministic and probabilistic modellers, their main problem is the lack of good quantitative data for infectious diseases. With some exceptions, infectious disease epidemiology has made rather few attempts to assess good numerical values for transmission rates, and figures for contact rates are even scarcer. Especially predictions will be very sensitive to exact numbers, and as a general rule one could say that it is much easier to write down the formulae of a model than to collect good data to put into it.

Summary

Models of diseases that spread person-to-person rely on the concept of reproduction rate, which is the average number of people infected by one case. This depends on the attack rate of the disease, on the frequency of contacts, and on the duration of infectivity. If the proportion immune in a group is high, few contacts will result in transmission, and epidemics will become impossible. This is called herd immunity.

A simple model for a childhood disease consists of three differential equations, and exhibits a few of the details characteristic of such a disease.

The major problem with all infectious disease models is that the contact pattern in the population is often unknown, and very complicated to model. This makes it exceedingly difficult to predict the future course of evolving epidemics.

In the following chapters we shall look at some examples where these specific concepts of infectious disease epidemiology have been studied.

References

1. Dietz K. Transmission and control of arbovirus diseases. In: Ludwig D, Cooke KL (eds) *Epidemiology*. Philadelphia: Society for Industrial and Applied Mathematics, 1975: 104–21.

11 Detection and analysis of outbreaks

Here the epidemiology of outbreak investigations is discussed. The importance of case definitions is stressed, and the various types of epidemic curves presented. Three examples of different outbreak investigations are dissected in some detail

Almost every investigation of an outbreak of a known or new disease starts with someone noticing an excess of cases. If you look back at Chapter 2, that is almost exactly the definition of an epidemic given by Benenson: 'The occurrence of cases of an illness clearly in excess of expectancy'. The key word here is 'expectancy': When does one get the feeling that this is more than it should have been? In the previous chapters, we have looked at the concepts of risks and rates from different angles, always stressing that such measures need not only a figure for the cases, but also some comparison or denominator. When someone suddenly notices an excess of cases, such formal comparisons are seldom made. Instead, one uses one's general, everyday knowledge and experience, which yield some rather imprecise feeling for what is usual and common and what is not.

Such notions are necessary for any more rigorous investigation to get started. However, one should be very careful not to put too much faith in them, and many misconceptions in medicine, and in human affairs in general, come from uncritical reliance on numbers, without considerations of denominators or control groups.

This concept of a perceived deviation from the normal can be carried over into the investigations of outbreaks. In such a situation, it is usually clear that something has happened outside 'expectancy'. The immediate task is to find and describe the cases, and to analyse them for any unexpected patterns. The controlling is supplied by common sense. If, for example, we find that 80% of the cases in an outbreak are women, this must be an important piece of information even without further formal analysis, since we know that the expected proportion should be around 50%. If we find that all the cases live in one section of a city, this is an unexpected finding, and would implicate some geographical risk of exposure. As an example of the inverse situation: a lack of outbreaks, Jenner noted in the late 1700s that milkmaids seldom fell ill with smallpox, and from this observation he proceeded to introduce vaccinia inoculation as a vaccine for smallpox.

Methods

Such an early analysis of an epidemiological pattern is sometimes called *descriptive* epidemiology. The three important words here are **time**, **place** and **person**, and the two questions that need to be answered as early as possible in an outbreak are:

1. What pathogen is causing the disease? and 2. Where is the source? However, even before these two questions are satisfactorily answered it may sometimes be possible to instigate broad preventive measures for the protection of the susceptible, such as recommending the boiling of drinking water, or closing a school.

The first thing one has to do is to decide who is a case and who is not. To this end, one needs a *case definition*, which should include the typical symptoms of the patients in the outbreak. Also, the time interval in which the illness should have broken out must be specified, because we do not want to include people with similar symptoms from other causes. A typical case definition could look like: 'All children in form 3 of the local school who took part in the field trip on November 20, and who fell ill with vomiting and/or diarrhoea between the evening of the 20th and the evening of the 21st.' The symptoms of the case definition are best assessed from interviews with a couple of cases regarded as typical of the outbreak. These people should also be the first ones to yield samples for microbiological analysis.

As you can see, such a rather detailed case definition already requires a quite good overview of the outbreak (group afflicted, times of onset), and often one does not have such a firm grip of the outbreak during the initial phases. It is best to start with a broad tentative definition, which can then be narrowed down as more and more about the outbreak becomes known.

During the following hours or days one tries to find all the cases of the outbreak, or at least a representative sample. Their sexes and ages should be recorded, as well as information on times of onset, symptoms, times of suspected exposures, and geographical information. If the disease is a gastroenteritis, one will try to get as detailed a food history as possible, if it is an airborne infection, one will need exact information on the patient's movements during the presumed incubation period.

It is almost always a good idea to develop a questionnaire before the interviews start. In this way, one will remember to ask all the pertinent questions, and if several different investigators are working simultaneously, a questionnaire will assure that they collect the same information.

The responses from the cases are used to make the following types of graphs:

Epidemic curve

The date at which each case fell ill is plotted along a horizontal axis in the following fashion, where each square denotes a patient as shown in Fig. 11.1. (One usually works from a list of cases, where each case has a number. It is often useful to write these numbers in the corresponding squares on the curve, since that will make it easy to go back and forth between the graph and the list).

No. of cases

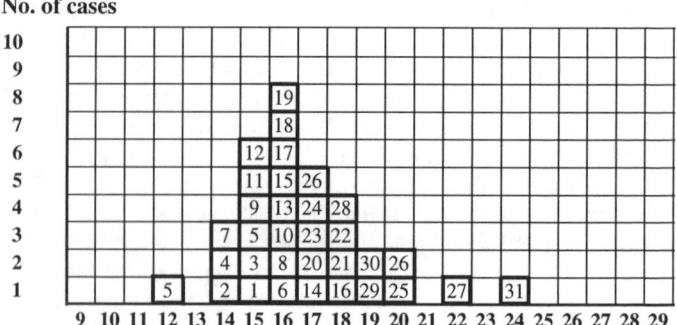

Fig. 11.1 An example of a point source outbreak.

In this particular epidemic, the earliest case happened on the 12th of the month, with incidence being highest on the 16th, and no case after the 24th. This type of epidemic curve, which is clustered around a peak value, points to a common event when all 31 cases were infected at the same time, and this is a typical example of a *point source outbreak.* You will notice that the first case to be diagnosed was not the first case in time. This is quite common in outbreak investigations, when extended case finding reveals cases that were not noticed, or not reported, initially.

Case 5 should correspond to the shortest possible incubation time for the disease, and case 31 to the longest. If we already have a suspect infectious event, we could guess which disease this is from knowledge of the incubation time of different diseases. Another type of epidemic curve is shown in Fig. 11.2 below.

No. of cases

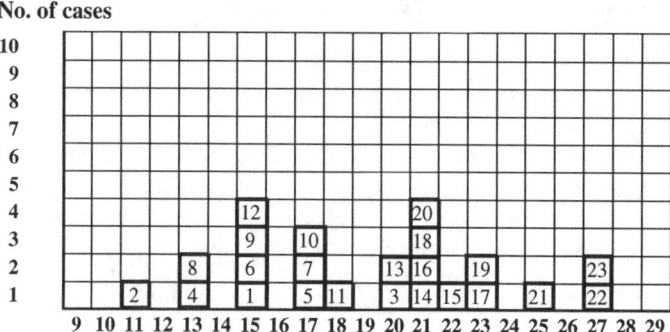

Fig. 11.2 An example of a continuous source outbreak.

Such a pattern is more indicative of a *continuous source,* where for example drinking water is being polluted, or some foodstuff is continuously contaminated.

In a person-to-person-spread situation, the epidemic curve will look like Fig. 11.3.

Here the person who fell ill on the 10th probably infected the group of people who fell ill between the 15th and 17th, and this group again caused a new group of cases around the 23rd. The interval between successive waves of disease seems to be around seven days, but you can see that the variation around this average value will make the cyclic epidemic pattern disappear after a couple of waves. As pointed out in Chapter 2, this interval is called the serial interval, and it is often shorter than the incubation period. This is evident if one considers that the index case could well have been infectious some days before he fell ill on the 10th, which means that the secondary cases had an incubation period of more than the five – eight days indicated by the above curve.

No. of cases

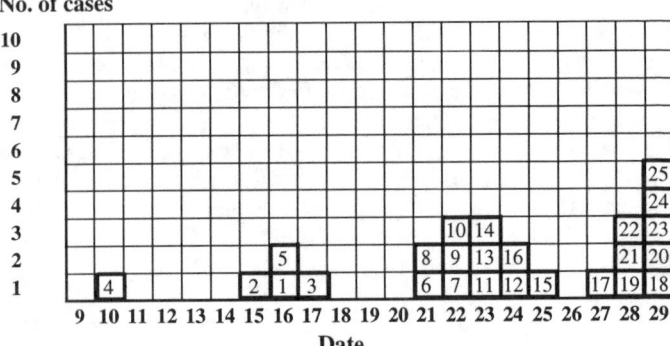

Date

Fig. 11.3 An example of a person-to-person spread (or propagated*) outbreak.*

Geography

In many outbreaks, it may be enlightening to plot all the cases on a map to see if there is evidence of clustering. In a modern society it is often quite difficult to decide which place should be plotted (home? work place? holiday resort?), since few people spend their days in the same place. In an outbreak of Legionnaires' disease in London in 1987, it could be shown that almost all the cases had visited an area downwind from a cooling tower in central London during the days when the bacteria were suspectedly spread.

Age and sex

A third plot that may yield information on aetiology is to draw a population pyramid of the cases. Fig. 11.4 is a rather extreme example, which builds on a real outbreak in Sweden several years ago.

This graph shows the different age groups going up, and the number of cases in each group as squares going left and right. The disease was a gastroenteritis, and there was a rather prolonged epidemic. What could cause this peculiar pattern, with cases among children, among young adult women, and among old people? (The answer is canned baby food, infected with salmonella. The babies obviously got it from eating baby food, their mothers from tasting before feeding them, and the old age pensioners from buying baby food for dental or economic reasons.)

All these curves only show the patterns among the cases, without any controls or denominators. However, as soon as we believe that we can see a pattern among the cases, we can go on to a more rigorous

Men   Women

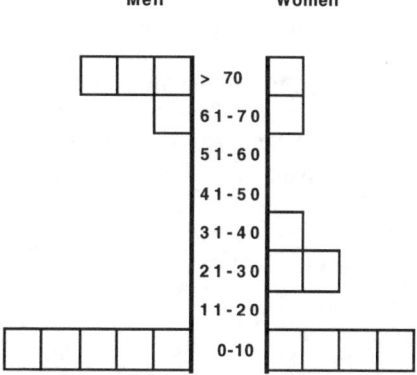

Fig. 11.4 *Simplified curve showing age and sex distribution of an outbreak of gastroenteritis in Sweden.*

analysis, by getting hold of those people who seem to have been exposed at the outbreak, but who did not fall ill. By asking those controls carefully about their exposures, it becomes possible to implicate a specific source much more reliably, just as we did in Chapters 3 and 4.

Three real-life examples

A hepatitis B outbreak

A good example of an outbreak investigation comes from a small epidemic of hepatitis B among diabetes patients in the USA.[1]

As always, the investigation was sparked by someone noticing an increased number of cases: during a ten-month period in 1989–90, 20 cases of acute hepatitis B were diagnosed among the patients in a hospital, compared to four during the previous year. This seems like a six-fold increase in incidence calculated on a yearly basis, provided that the denominator remained constant, i.e. constant rates of admissions and discharges during the two periods.

The 20 patients during the 10-month period were initially defined as the cases, and their medical records sought for possible connections. It was found that 18 of them had diabetes, that all but one were male, and that they had all been admitted to one single medical ward at some time during the six months preceding their illness. Common sense is enough to decide that it is improbable that these three findings should have arisen by chance.

The next step was to look actively for more cases. All of the more than 500 patients who had been admitted to the ward at any time during 1989 and who were still alive at the time of the study were approached and requested to provide a blood sample. Seven more cases were detected this way. An interesting point mentioned in the paper is that only seven of the 27 cases (26%) had any symptoms of an acute hepatitis B infection. There must have been a continuing strategy of testing for hepatitis markers in this hospital, or the outbreak would hardly have been discovered.

The resulting epidemic curve for the entire 14-month outbreak is shown in Fig. 11.5.

No. of cases

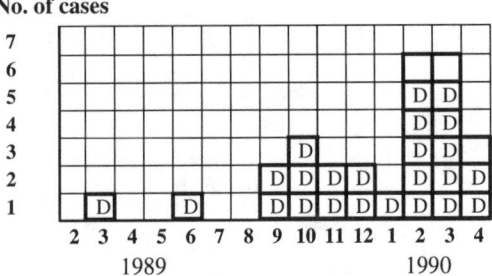

Fig. 11.5 *Epidemic curve for a prolonged outbreak of hepatitis B on a ward. D represents diabetes patients.* Source: *Polish* et al.[1]

The incubation period of hepatitis B is two to six months, and the serial interval perhaps one month shorter. The epidemic curve could thus describe a person-to-person spread, with the primary case being diagnosed in March 1989, the secondary case diagnosed in June 1989, and 25 tertiary and higher-order cases thereafter.

The risk factors for becoming infected (other than having diabetes) were explored in a retrospective cohort study, including all patients with diabetes who had been admitted to the ward after the primary case above had been discharged. Twenty-three of them were the cases in Fig. 11.5, and 37 were still susceptible to hepatitis B infection. Relative risk for becoming infected was calculated for a number of factors, such as age, sex, race, date of hospitalization, location of beds in the ward, other behavioural risks, etc. The only factor that showed a strong association with infection was the use of a spring-loaded device for taking capillary blood samples, for which the 2 × 2 table became:

	Spring device used	Not used	
Infected	23	0	23
Susceptible	32	5	37
	55	5	60

The risk of infection in the patients who had samples taken with the spring-loaded device was thus $23/55 = 0.42$, versus $0/5 = 0$ in the group who had not had their capillary samples taken in this way. The probability that this difference would occur by chance is 0.08, according to Fisher's exact test.

The investigators then proceeded to perform a case-control study, comparing the three nondiabetic patients who contracted hepatitis with a random sample of 20 nondiabetic, still susceptible patients from the population of all patients who had been hospitalized during the year. When analysing for the exposure 'having had capillary test taken by spring-loaded device', they got the following result:

	Spring device used	Not used	
Infected	3	0	3
Susceptible	0	20	20
	3	20	23

The OR cannot be calculated, due to the zeros, but Fisher's exact test gives the probability that all the three infected patients should have been exposed to this risk, versus none of the 20 others just by chance to be 0.006.

The authors conclude that minute amounts of infected blood could have remained on the device, which was used consecutively on patients, and that this was the probable source of infection. The first case above was a hepatitis B carrier, and the second was a long-term patient of the ward, who was tested for capillary blood glucose regularly, and who could have acted as a 'reservoir' for the spread to other patients.

Lyme disease and ticks

A more protracted example of an outbreak investigation, and one which concerned a new disease, comes from the analysis of early data on Lyme disease:[2] this investigation started in 1975, when some mothers observed that a high number of children in a small, rural area of Connecticut were diagnosed as having juvenile rheumatoid

arthritis, which is usually a rare disease. This observation was followed by a retrospective analysis of 51 cases in the area in early
1976. On four country roads, one child in 10 had the disease, and in
that area there were six families who had had more than one case.

Quite early in the investigations, suspicion was directed towards
arthropod bites as the aetiology of the disease, and especially tick
bites. A prospective study was initiated to run through 1977, which
tried to collect all cases of Lyme disease diagnosed in an area of 12
communities on both sides of the Connecticut River.

All physicians and visiting nurses in the area were asked to report cases to the investigators at Yale University, and if possible to
refer the patients to them. No laboratory test for the disease was
available at the time, so the case definition was entirely clinical,
based on the appearance of a typical exanthema, or on brief but
recurrent aseptic arthritis.

Forty-three patients were reported during the year. There was of
course no way to ascertain the completeness of the reporting, but 41
of the 55 participating physicians reported at least one case. A chart
plotting the epidemic is shown in Fig. 11.6.

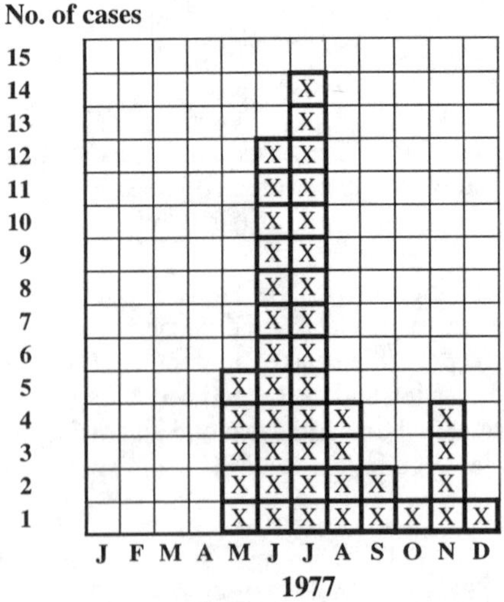

No. of cases

Fig. 11.6 *Epidemic curve for an outbreak of Lyme disease in Connecticut,
1977.* Source: *Steere* et al.[2]

The cases start appearing in May, incidence peaks in early summer,
and there are still cases diagnosed during the autumn. The months

of June and July are responsible for 60% of the cases.

The most striking finding appeared when the patients were divided into those living east and west of the Connecticut River: there were 35 cases on the east side, and only eight on the west side. In order to assess the value of this information, we need denominators. If there were many more people living on the east side, this could explain the difference in numbers. However, there were 12,400 residents in the communities on the east side, and 60,300 on the west side. The risks of disease during the year were thus 2.8 and 0.13 per 1000 residents, respectively. The relative risk can be calculated to be 21, and an approximate 95% confidence interval is obtained from the formula in Chapter 5. The error factor would be:

$$EF = e^{2\sqrt{1/a+1/b}}$$

where $a = 35$ and $b = 8$ (both figures should really be greater than 10 for the formula to be quite valid, but we will just get a rough estimate here),

$$EF = e^{2\sqrt{1/8+1/35}} = 2.2$$

and the lower limit is thus $21/2.2 = 9.5$, which is well above unity.

The sex relationship of the cases was 1.2 to 1, men to women, so this did not yield much additional information. Half the cases were in children aged 15 or younger, and only one patient was older than 50.

All the findings so far presented fit in rather nicely with the hypothesis of an arthropod vector (and especially a non-flying one): the incidence curve correlates well with the life cycle of arthropods, the geographical division by the river could be explained by differing densities of the vector, and the excess of cases in children could be due to the fact that they spend more time out of doors. However, there are many possible biases to be considered:

1. Seasonal variations in incidence are seen for many diseases, and, for example, dietary habits or amounts of allergens in the environment could well vary to cause patterns similar to the one in the curve above.
2. The geographical difference could be due to increased clinical awareness in the doctors on the east side of the river.
3. There could be genetic differences between the populations on either side of the river.
4. The age pattern could be due to worried parents consulting physicians for symptoms in their children, but disregarding similar symptoms in themselves.

Next, the investigators performed a case-control study. For each of the 32 patients who were diagnosed between June and September, two neighbourhood controls were chosen, matched on sex and on child/adult. (It is not clear from the article why controls were not selected for all the cases.) The cases and controls were interviewed about a list of possible risk factors, such as the size of their plot, types of outside activities, pets and farm animals, and recollection of arthropod bites in 1977.

Significantly more cases reported tick bites than did the controls. The former also reported having seen ticks on their pet animals more often than the later. Even this finding could be due to confounding: if the real risk factor was something else that one would encounter in the wild, then the group of people who reported a tick bite would probably contain a higher proportion of people who spent much time out of doors, and who would thus run a higher risk of being exposed to the real risk factor. The tick bite would then be a marker of risk behaviour, and not the real cause.

At the same time as this investigation was performed, however, another group measured the density of the tick *Ixodes scapularis* east and west of the river, and found it to be about 15 times more prevalent on wild animals on the east side.[3] All this pointed to an aetiological role for bites from this tick, and a few years later the spirochaete *Borrelia burgdorferi* was isolated from these ticks and found to be related to a number of clinical symptoms in humans.

Legionnaire's disease

On July 21–24, 1976, the American Legion, Department of Pennsylvania (a congregation of war veterans), held a convention in a hotel in Philadelphia. The 2 August, it became clear that there was an outbreak of severe pneumonia of unknown aetiology among the participants, and the Pennsylvania Department of Health started an investigation.[4] A case was defined as someone who had:
- either attended the convention, or
- who had entered the hotel after July 1,

and who had onset between July 1 and August 18
- cough and fever $\geq 38.9°$ C, or
- any fever and X-ray verified pneumonia.

One can see that the clinical case definition is rather wide, and that it probably will include pneumonias of other aetiologies. Also, the time period in the epidemiological case definition starts well before the known outbreak, to make certain that early cases were not missed, something that would be particularly important if the disease was spread person-to-person and had an incubation period in the order of weeks.

Cases were sought actively over the entire state of Pennsylvania, public health nurses searching hospitals for hospitalized participants, and the public being invited to report cases on a telephone hot line. Altogether 182 patients meeting the case definition were found, 29 of whom died from the disease for a case-fatality rate of 16%. One hundred and forty-nine had attended the convention, and another nine had attended other conventions in the hotel just before of just after the Legionnaires' meeting. Eighty-four of the patients had stayed at least one night in the hotel. Figure 11.7 illustrates the epidemic curve.

Cases

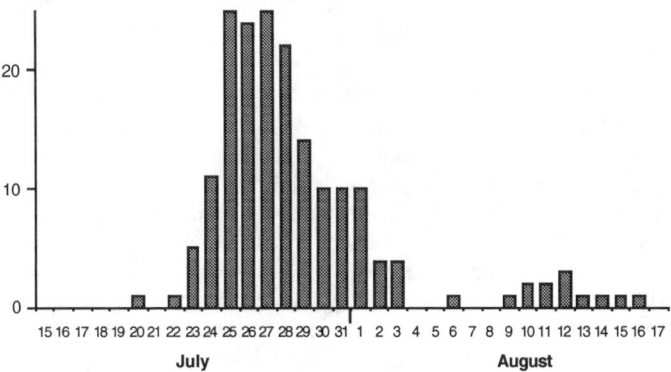

Fig. 11.7 Epidemic curve for the outbreak in which Legionnaire's disease was first described. Source: *Fraser* et al.[4]

Disregarding the trickle of cases in August, this epidemic curve almost looks like a textbook example of a point source outbreak.

There was no evidence of similar outbreaks connected to other hotels in the area during the time, nor of any general increase in pneumonia mortality in Pennsylvania. There were, however, 39 additional patients found, who met the clinical criteria, and who had been within one block of the hotel (but not entered) during the time period of the case definition.

One hundred and forty-two cases (78%) were men, which is not surprising since this was a veteran's meeting. For the same reason, the age distribution was rather skew towards higher ages.

This is the straightforward time-place-person description of the outbreak. However, the significance of the right-skewed age distribution cannot be assessed since we do not know the age distribution of all people who came to the convention. The investigators tried to distribute a questionnaire to all participants, and received a reply from 84%. From these forms they could calculate age-specific attack rates (bringing in a denominator!), which are shown in Table 11.1.

Table 11.1 *Attack rate by age during an outbreak of Legionnaire's disease.* Source: *Fraser* et al.[4]

Age group	Cases	Total	Attack rate (%)
< 40	6	160	3.8
40–49	20	392	5.1
50–59	52	843	6.2
60–69	31	315	9.8
≥ 70	16	130	12.3
Total	125	1849	6.8

The attack rate evidently increased with age. It was also higher for delegates than for other people attending the convention.

If 'visiting the hotel' was taken as the time of exposure, the incubation time for all but two cases could be estimated to be between two and 10 days.

On the 17 August a telephone interview was undertaken with 113 cases and 147 controls. The subjects were asked about their movements during the four days, and since cases had occurred among people who did not even enter the hotel, the subjects were asked to specify how much time they had spent in the lobby or on the pavement outside the hotel.

Fifty percent of the cases resided in the convention hotel, versus only 35% of the controls. This difference was significant. Furthermore, the cases had spent almost twice as many minutes in the lobby, on average, as had the controls. Among the persons who watched the Legion parade on the 23 July, cases were more likely than controls to have stood on the sidewalk directly in front of the hotel.

The possibility of person-to-person spread was also examined in a case-control study: 59 room mates of 52 cases were compared with 69 room mates of 68 controls. Five room mates from each group (8.5 and 7.2%, respectively) were themselves taken ill. The difference is small and statistically nonsignificant, and shows that person-to-person spread was unlikely. Neither were any relatives of cases infected after their return home.

All this evidence pointed to an airborne agent for this infection, which must have been most abundant in the lobby and directly outside the hotel. In fact, simultaneously with this investigation, the bacteria *Legionella* was being isolated in the laboratory, and a serological test for infection was also used in the epidemiological work.

Summary

The three important factors to be characterized in an outbreak analysis are time, place and person. In order to identify the cases for this analysis, one needs a case definition, and this is used to actively search for more cases than the ones who presented themselves. The epidemic curve can give indication on type of exposure: point source, extended source, or person-to-person. In a point source outbreak it is often possible to estimate the common time of exposure, if the disease and its incubation time are known, or conversely, diagnose the disease if time of exposure is known.

Plots should be made not only for time course of the outbreak, but also for sex and age distribution, and often for the geographical location of the cases.

After the cases have been identified, the probable cause of the outbreak can be searched by more analytical methods, most often starting with a case-control study. In many instances, the cause will be clear from the outset, since an unexpected increase in rate of diagnosis of a certain pathogen in the microbiological laboratory will often be what triggered the investigation. However, if the pathogen was previously unknown, epidemiology and microbiology must often work hand in hand to reveal the cause.

References

1. Polish LB, Shapiro CN, Bauer F *et al*. Nosocomial transmission of hepatitis B virus associated with the use of a spring-loaded finger-stick device. *N Engl J Med* 1992: **326**; 721–25.

2. Steere AC, Broderick TF, Malawista SE. Erythema chronicum migrans and Lyme arthritis: epidemiologic evidence for a tick vector. *Am J Epidemiol* 1978; **108**: 312–21.

3. Wallis RC, Brown SE, Kloter KO, Main AJ. Erythema chronicum migrans and Lyme arthritis: field study of ticks. *Am J Epidemiol* 1978; **108**: 322–27.

4. Fraser DW, Tsai TR, Orenstein W, *et al*. Legionnaire's disease. Description of an epidemic of pneumonia. *N Engl J Med* 1977; **297**: 1189–97.

12 Routine surveillance of infectious diseases

This chapter discusses how data for surveillance is collected and interpreted. Several sources of potential bias are identified.

The previous chapter described the analysis of outbreaks of known or new diseases. In each example the discovery of the outbreak relied on clinical observations, where an unusual aggregation of cases was first noted by physicians or the public. This is a somewhat haphazard mode of detection, and at least for known diseases with an epidemic potential one would feel more secure with an established system that could recognize outbreaks when they occurred.

Since the end of last century, many Western countries have thus had systems for the reporting ('notification') of certain infectious diseases. There is also mandatory reporting to the World Health Organization of cases of cholera, yellow fever, or plague in any of its member countries. The aim of such reporting systems has always been to quickly discover epidemic outbreaks of infectious disease, and the rationale is that while any one doctor might only see one or two cases of an epidemic, the collected reporting to the regional or national level will make it possible to see the full picture.

These notification systems were not instituted as a purely epidemiological exercise, but rather to make possible the rapid application of preventive measures. Exactitude is therefore often less important than speed, and there is seldom time for elaborate epidemiological analysis of data before an action is decided on.

This continuous collection, collation and analysis of data, with or without subsequent action, is often called *surveillance*. A large part of studies on infectious disease epidemiology emanate from such surveillance data.

The general principle is that each country has a list of notifiable diseases, which may vary in length from around 10 to over 50 in European countries. Each time a physician diagnoses a patient with one of these diseases, he should report this to the regional or national level. This notification usually goes by mail, but electronic networks are coming more and more into use. The amount of information on the notification form varies greatly between countries, but most often includes diagnosis, date of onset, age, sex, and residence of the patient. It may also contain data on symptoms, type of exposure, other similar cases in the vicinity, and on treatment given and precautions taken.

Another way of collecting incidence data is by reports from the microbiological laboratories. Since for many of the notifiable diseases diagnosis is now confirmed by microbiological analysis, a standardized reporting from these laboratories will include most such cases. With more and more laboratories computerizing the handling of samples and reports, such notification could soon also be by direct electronic transmission.

A third data source are discharge notes from hospitals, which should include diagnoses and some data about the patients. The main problems with this source are that it will only contain the most severe cases of the disease (those who were hospitalized), and that the time lag from admittance to reporting is often long in a routine system.

The main task of a surveillance system is to discover sudden changes in incidence, i.e. outbreaks or epidemics. In such situations it becomes important that the system's sensitivity for detecting cases is high. This sensitivity may be the sum of several factors, such as the clinician's diagnostic accuracy, microbiological test methods, reporting propensity, etc. On the other hand, specificity need not be so high; it is of little consequence if a few cases too many are reported in an epidemic situation.

Such surveillance of incidence cannot be restricted to overall figures for a nation, it must also look at regional differences. An increased incidence in one part of a country may be masked by decreasing incidence somewhere else, keeping the total constant. In short, a surveillance system looks for *clusters* of disease, in time and in space.

There is, however, a need for a note of caution concerning surveillance data: Increasingly, such data are being used for other purposes than cluster alert. They are utilized to monitor long term trends, to make international comparisons, and to analyse costs and benefits of preventive measures. Such uses put quite new demands on the quality of the data, and on the stringency of the epidemiological analysis. This has given national and regional surveillance units in several countries a new role, having to switch from outbreak investigations to more subtle analyses – a change with which some of them are still grappling.

Discovering outbreaks

There are no simple rules of thumb to decide when an outbreak is under way; just as with the word 'epidemic', definitions are difficult. For many diseases, such as salmonella, gonorrhoea, or measles there will be a steady trickle of cases notified, and the task is to see when this endemic situation is replaced by an outbreak. Other diseases such as plague or rabies are sufficiently rare in Western countries to warrant an outbreak investigation after just one case.

Because for many diseases there will always be a number of expected cases reported each week, surveillance implies continuous comparison of actual number of cases with the expected. In a conscientious surveillance programme, even minor deviations should at least be noted and given a second thought, although this second thought may lead to the decision not to do anything. What constitutes a minor as opposed to an alerting deviation is very much a question of experience, and in most national or regional surveillance units there will be written and unwritten standards for action. In all such units there will always have been instances of heightened vigilance in response to suspected outbreaks, which were subsequently disregarded, and never reached public attention.

Even though the aim of a notification system is to give the central agency power to detect outbreaks, many outbreaks are in reality first detected by astute clinicians. The best example from recent time is the discovery of AIDS: in the summer of 1981 two groups of clinicians in the USA almost simultaneously reported on an unexpected incidence of strange diseases in young homosexual men: pneumonia caused by *Pneumocystis carinii* in Los Angeles[1] and the skin tumour Kaposi's sarcoma in New York.[2] The US central agency Centers for Disease Control in Atlanta immediately reacted to those reports, and started a surveillance scheme, which finally led to the description of the new disease, but the original observation was made by clinicians.

Analysing outbreaks

Once an outbreak has been established, the normal, 'passive' surveillance relying on notifications is often replaced by a more active
phase, in which investigators are sent to the afflicted area to collect
more information, much as described in the previous chapter. However, since a routine surveillance system is devised to detect changes
in incidence of a number of listed diseases, the specific cause is
usually known for outbreaks noted at the central level, and the
investigation will focus on possible sources.

The need to cover a greater geographical area is evident from,
for example, the present food distribution patterns of most countries, where an infected sending of foodstuff may be distributed over
wide areas, and where sporadic cases may appear in many different
places, without being recognized as parts of an outbreak. A good
example comes from a contamination of chocolate bars with salmonella in the UK in the early 1980s:[3]

During May 1982, three cases of infection with *Salmonella napoli*
were reported to the Communicable Disease Surveillance Centre.
Because there had only been 15 cases diagnosed in the UK during
the 30 previous years, this incidence was higher than expected:
calculated as yearly incidence it would correspond to 36 cases,
compared with the expected 0.5. Twenty-nine additional cases were
reported in June.

The investigation started with telephone interviews and visits to
determine date of onset, geographical distribution and age/sex of
the patients. It became clear that most cases lived in south east England, and that children below the age of 15 were in majority.

Quite early, the investigators started to suspect a brand of
imported chocolate bars. In early July, they performed a small case-
control study, where they collected food histories for the week preceding the illness from 17 patients. In order to investigate exposures
in an outbreak like this, it is very important that secondary cases,
infected by someone else in the family, are not included. Such cases
may not have had the exposure one is trying to assess, and adding
them will introduce a misclassification, which will weaken the
strength of any association found. Therefore, one has to be quite
careful when ascertaining dates of onset, and one also needs knowledge of the incubation times of salmonella infections.

Twenty-four controls were chosen by asking the patients or their
parents to name a household in the neighbourhood with people in
the same age groups, or just by randomly approaching a neighbouring

house. The controls were asked about food consumption during the week preceding the illness in the corresponding case. Note the choice of time period here: in order to get adequate control data it would not be appropriate to ask the controls what they ate during the last week. They must be asked about exposures during exactly the time period as the cases were presumably exposed.

The 2 × 2 table for this first case-control study looked like:

	Case	Neighbour	
Ate chocolate bar	9	0	9
Did not eat	8	24	32
	17	24	41

Over half of the cases had eaten (or remembered that they had eaten) chocolate bars, versus none of the controls. Since there is a zero in the top right-hand cell, we cannot calculate an odds ratio (it would be infinite), but using Fisher's exact test we find that the probability that the cases and controls would have these patterns of chocolate consumption just by chance is less than 0.0001.

This investigation led to the recall of the chocolate bars from all shops from late July, but during July and first half of August more cases were diagnosed, and extended collection of faecal samples also revealed a number of asymptomatic carriers. Fifty-eight percent of the cases were below 15 years of age, and of the older cases 60% were women. The geographical analysis showed that during the first months, almost all the cases came from south-east England, where the chocolate bars were first marketed, whilst during the latter half of the outbreak, most of the cases were from northern England, where sales started in late June. The final case-control study included 93 cases and 122 controls, and looked like:

	Case	Neighbour	
Ate chocolate bar	57	3	60
Did not eat	36	119	155
	93	122	215

The OR for chocolate bars was $(57/36)/(3/119) = 62.8$, with a 95% confidence interval from 18.5 to 213, which is comfortably above 1. There thus seems to have been a strong association between disease and chocolate bar consumption.

Another example of the need of national, or even international, surveillance comes from outbreaks of Legionnaire's disease in holiday travellers from northern Europe to Mediterranean resorts. In several instances *Legionella* was being spread from hotel air conditioning systems or showers, and some tourists became ill upon returning home. The number of cases detected in each country may have been very small, but by combining data from the different home countries of tourists that had stayed in the same hotel, it became possible to elucidate the cause of the outbreak and to instigate preventive measures.

Validity of notification data

The most important problem in the interpretation of notification data concerns their validity – do they really measure what we want them to measure? Is the yearly number of notified cases of a certain disease equal to the incidence? Can observed changes over time be safely interpreted to represent changes in the underlying incidence rate?

The number of patients reported with a certain disease will be influenced by many factors that may well change over time or between places, and this will create biases when comparisons are made. Some such factors are:

1. Attendance patterns

People's propensity to seek medical care can not be assumed to be constant. The distance to the nearest hospital or clinic will play a role, as will costs and waiting times. Media reports of an outbreak will always bring more people to the clinic, and a portion of these will probably have milder infections, which would not ordinarily have made them come. Public awareness will thus increase observed incidence.

2. Diagnostic methods

Obviously, new tests that make it possible to diagnose atypical or asymptomatic cases of a disease will lead to an increased reported incidence. A rather nice example comes from the introduction of chlamydia cultures in Sweden in the late 1970s (see Fig. 12.1).

There seemed to be a substantial increase in incidence of chlamydia infections during the first part of the decade, with a doubling of cases from 1983 to 1987. However, what happened was that more and more of the microbiological laboratories started to set up chlamydia testing and making it available to the clinicians during this time. By plotting the total number of cultures performed each year we get the following picture (Fig. 12.2).

Reported cases

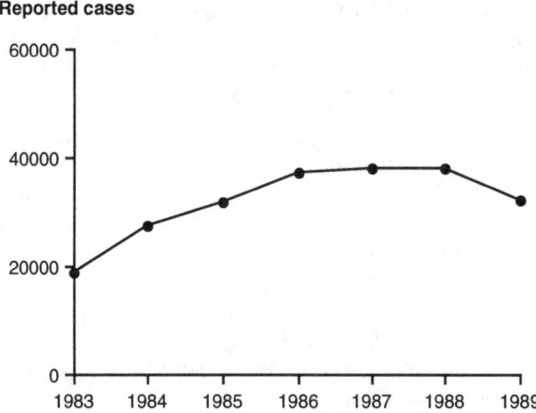

Fig. 12.1 *Laboratory reported cases of genital chamydia infection in Sweden in 1983–1989.*

The graph below shows an almost perfect parallel increase in samples taken and patients diagnosed between 1983 and 1986. Each year, one tenth of the samples turned out positive. Therefore, the apparent epidemic of chlamydia was most likely due to improved diagnostic facilities, and not to an increased transmission. There is no reason to believe that there were fewer cases in 1980 than in 1987; we just could not find them at that time. (Additionally, one

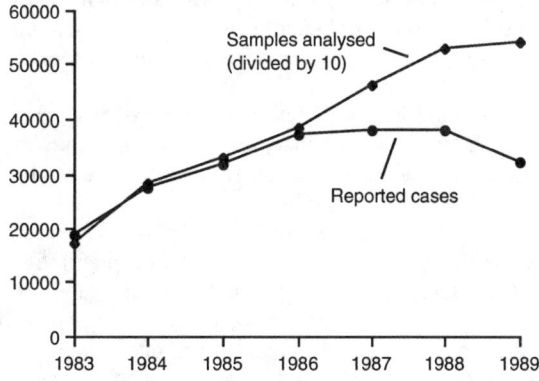

Fig. 12.2 *Same graph as in Fig. 12.1, but also including number of samples analysed each year (divided by 10 to get the scales equal).*

can see that after 1988 the number of reported cases started to decrease whilst testing was still increasing, which supports the suspicion that there has been a real decrease in incidence after that time.)

3. Screening

A related problem comes from the setting up of screening programmes for asymptomatic infections. Such programmes will always lead to an apparent increase in incidence: 'Seek, and ye shall find.' This situation is, however, quite far removed from the original surveillance model, where sick people came to the doctor and were diagnosed.

In order to separate the cases found through screening from the symptomatic ones, notification forms now sometimes contain a question about why the test was done: patient's initiative, clinical suspicion, screening, etc. In my experience it is often difficult for a doctor to specify this precisely; there may be several factors behind the decision to perform a test, and the request to single out one is often artificial.

4. Reporting propensity

Even though many countries have statutory notification of a number of diseases, the adherence to such rules varies enormously between them. Comparison between countries of figures published in national statistics is for the most part meaningless unless one has good information on the notification completeness behind those figures. Generally, notification works better in countries with a nationalized health care system than in countries with many independent clinics and laboratories.

Also within countries, notification percentages may vary, and doctors often show a similar behaviour as patients: when there is increased media awareness of a certain disease, those cases become diagnosed and notified more readily.

The four above points are all examples of biases (a term for this type of bias would be *assessment bias*) that could enter notification data, and they underline the caution with which such data should be approached. Does this mean that such surveillance systems fill no useful purpose? No, not necessarily, as long as one remembers their original raison d'être, which is to discover sudden changes in incidence for a number of listed diseases. To this end, it does not matter if only a portion of all physicians report their cases as long as this portion is roughly constant over time. If, for example, a steady 15% of the doctors in a country are careful about sending in their notifications, incidence changes on a national scale will be detected anyhow. Also, the other sources of bias listed above will tend to be less problematic when the time scale is short.

There is also another, somewhat philosophical, problem connected to the use of notification data to describe routes of transmission. Let us take the example of infection with *Campylobacter pylori* and chicken consumption in Sweden: not long after the bacteria was first described, it was found to be part of the normal intestinal flora of many birds. There were also some early reports of small family outbreaks of campylobacter diarrhoea after eating undergrilled chicken. The connection between chicken and this infection soon became well known to most clinicians, and they started asking their campylobacter patients if they had eaten chicken during the week or so before onset. As it is, chicken is a very common food in Sweden, and a high proportion of the patients would answer 'yes', even though the chicken they ate might have had nothing to do with their disease. On the notification form, the clinician would put 'eaten chicken' in the box for possible risk factors. A large number of the forms on campylobacter enteritis received at the national surveillance institute would thus have chicken as most probable source, and in next year's annual report it would stand out as the most common risk factor. This would in turn even further increase the clinicians' awareness of this route of infection, which would lead even more of them to ask about chicken consumption, and so on. This example points to the intrinsic 'conservative' nature of notification systems, especially if the risk comes from an exposure that is common, but only rarely the cause of disease. Most physicians will feel quite content when their interview with the patient has revealed one established risk factor, and in situations like these, a notification system may tend to overestimate the importance of this factor and instead fail to detect other important routes of transmission.

Notification delays

There will always be a delay between diagnosis of a case and the arrival of the notification form at the central surveillance agency. This obviously has consequences for prevention, and you will find that the majority of reported point source outbreaks in the literature had actually subsided well before they were detected.

Reporting delays may also have statistical implications. Published surveillance statistics usually date cases by the day the form was received, not by actual date of diagnosis or of onset. Cases diagnosed late in one year may thus be registered the following year. A curve showing, for example, weekly incidence over one year may indicate low incidence during holiday periods: when staff are short and everyone is too busy to fill out notification forms, and then a notable peak when all the forms were mailed at the same time. Such a peak could easily deceive a novice reader that there had been a real epidemic just after the holiday period.

The issue of notification delays is quite important for surveillance, but it has not received much attention. One exception is a study from the UK in 1987,[4] which used the information on notification slips to estimate the time from diagnosis to receipt of the form for 15 different diseases. Delay was found to vary by region and by disease, being five days on average for measles but more than two months for tuberculosis. It also seemed to be increasing during the study period. However, it was not until the emergence of the AIDS epidemic that notification delays were studied more systematically. Accurate knowledge of past incidence is critical for projections on the future size of the epidemic. Firstly, it was found in several Western countries that some 10–20% of all cases were never notified. Secondly, even for notified cases there were often long delays, so that typically only 80% were reported in the year of diagnosis, and some cases still being reported two or more years after they had first been diagnosed. The pattern of this reporting delay has been studied in several countries, and it has to be corrected for in models on future AIDS incidence.

Feedback of information

The probably most important part of a surveillance system that builds on the active participation of a large number of physicians is information feedback: if the central agency just collects the data and analyses it, but fails to report back relevant findings to the people in the field, their interest in reporting will wane. They must feel that the information they get in return for spending time filling out forms is relevant to them in their daily work with patients. Adequate and timely information could aid in making diagnoses, choosing treatments, and also in increasing vigilance for specific diseases.

You will find solemn declarations like the above paragraph in any text on surveillance, but proper feedback is a difficult task. In most epidemic situations it has to be rapid, because there is little use in being told about an epidemic that has already subsided. It also has to be clinically relevant, which is why it is important that the people responsible for the dissemination of the collated information keep a constant contact with the physicians who are the recipients.

Other data sources

Active surveillance cannot only rely on notifications, it must make use of all available sources. These include laboratory reports, informal contacts with colleagues, media items, and sometimes even rumours. Often, a more active role must be assumed, where clinicians are approached directly and asked about suspect cases. In a recent study of such a serious disease as paralytic poliomyelitis in England, only nine out of 19 finally analysed cases had been notified, the others were found along other routes.[5] Obviously, however, the more one departs from a standardized data collection scheme, the less certain can one be of the representativity of the data.

Summary

Surveillance is an important part of practical infectious disease epidemiology. It builds on the notion that whilst any physician may only see one or two cases of an epidemic, and thus not be aware of it, the collected notifications on a regional or national level will make it possible to see the whole picture.

Active cooperation is required between clinicians and some central surveillance agency, where both parts should benefit from the activity. Rapid dissemination of analysed data back to the original suppliers in a fashion that they find useful in their daily work is the most important component; a system where the periphery feeds data into the centre without seeing any practical result is bound to falter.

References

1. Centers for Disease Control. *Pneumocystis pneumonia* – Los Angeles. *Morb Mort Weekly Rep* 1981; **30**: 250–52.

2. Centers for Disease Control. Kaposi's sarcoma and pneumocystis pneumonia among homosexual men – New York City and California. *Morb Mort Weekly Rep* 1981; **30**: 305–308.

3. Gill ON, Bartlett CLR, Sockett PN, et al. Outbreak of *Salmonella napoli* infection caused by contaminated chocolate bars. *Lancet* 1983; **1**: 574–77.

4. Clarkson JA, Fine PEM. Delays in notification of infectious disease. *Health Trends* 1987; **19**: 9–11.

5. Joyce R, Wood D, Brown D, Begg N. Paralytic poliomyelitis in England and Wales, 1985-91. *Br Med J* 1992; **305**: 79–82.

13 Measuring infectivity

We study how to answer the probably most common question regarding infectious diseases: 'How infectious is it?'. Different definitions of attack rate are discussed with some published examples of studies. The importance of dose and immunity is exemplified, and the subclinical infections are not forgotten.

One of the most important objectives for infectious disease epidemiology is obviously to measure infectivity. This is often quite difficult. One problem is that meaning of this term is not well defined in most instances. Another is that infectivity may vary with different external factors, for example, it may be quite different in different types of contacts between an infectious and a susceptible individual, as pointed out in Chapter 10. A third problem when measuring infectivity for a disease that is spread person-to-person, is to be certain that one part is infectious and the other susceptible at the time of their contact.

Part of the semantic problem comes from lack of reflection over the concept 'risk of becoming infected'. My risk of coming down with influenza during the next epidemic depends on two different factors:

1. The probability that I meet someone who is infectious with influenza. This probability is in its turn dependent on overall prevalence as well as on my contact pattern with people.
2. The risk that the virus is transmitted when I meet someone who is infectious. This risk in turn depends on how close our contact is.

A third factor influencing the risk is that I may be immune to the strain responsible for the next epidemic, but we will disregard that here.

Of the two first factors above, only the second has to do with infectivity. Any numerical value given for infectivity (or attack rate) will, however, have to be accompanied by a definition of the type of contact to which it applies.

The basic assumption in all calculations of attack rates is that the people in the denominator were really exposed to the pathogen. There is seldom any way of really ascertaining this, and it becomes a question of common sense and probabilities. For airborne infections it depends on proximity, wind directions and the volume of the space where the index case and the exposed were congregated.

With foodborne infections it should be realized that the pathogen may not be evenly distributed within the food. A pie that has been infected with a few *Salmonella* bacteria and left at room temperature some time before it is to be consumed may show large variations in the number of bacteria per bite.

When studying the effect of condom usage on risk of STD transmission, one must take several factors into account: was the condom used during the entire intercourse? Did it break? Could fingers have transferred the infection?

A recent issue has been to estimate the risk of sexual transmission of hepatitis C virus, and different studies have come to quite conflicting results. The problem has mainly been the lack of tests to ascertain whether the index person is really infectious. Serology shows whether or not a person has been infected with the virus, but not whether he is still transmitting it.

Examples – household infections

One of the best studies of infectivity performed was the one by Hope Simpson already mentioned in Chapter 3. He wanted to measure the attack rates of measles, chickenpox and mumps,[1] being well aware of the above problems. The design was as described below.

First he observed that 'the epidemic pattern depends in part on the natural characters of the parasite, in part on the human host'. He went on to say that he wanted to eliminate any disturbing influence of human behaviour on his measurements, or stated in modern epidemiological jargon: he wanted to control for differences in contact patterns. This he achieved by looking only at transmission within households. The study was undertaken in a part of Gloucestershire between 1947 and 1951, and aimed at collecting data on all exposures and transmissions of these three diseases in households in the area. The assumption he made is obviously that the contact pattern, and thus risk of exposure to a case, was sufficiently similar in all the families to justify the calculation of average values across households.

The exact method of ascertaining the index cases is not described in his article, and one must assume that they were the children who were diagnosed by the local GPs. After a case had been diagnosed, a member of the epidemiological research unit visited this household several times, checking up on the contacts. This method should be described as active surveillance, where cases are actually sought, and not only routinely reported. The parents were also carefully asked whether any of the other children had had this disease before.

All susceptible siblings then constitute a cohort, in which the risk of disease after contact with an index case can be calculated. The members of this cohort enter the study at different dates during a four-year period, but since risk of transmission should be the same in 1947 as in 1951, each sibling's time in the study can be regarded as starting on the day when the index case fell ill.

A general problem with studies of transmission in households concerns counting the number of exposures. In families with only two children it is easy, the sibling who is not the primary case is only exposed once. However, if there are three children or more, matters can become complicated. Suppose there are five children in a family: A, B, C, D and E. A is a primary case, and infects B, but C, D and E escape the first round. Then B infects C, but D and E still remain susceptible. In this family there were thus two transmissions, but what is the number of exposures? One way of counting would be to list the number of susceptibles exposed to every new generation of cases as shown in Fig. 13.1.

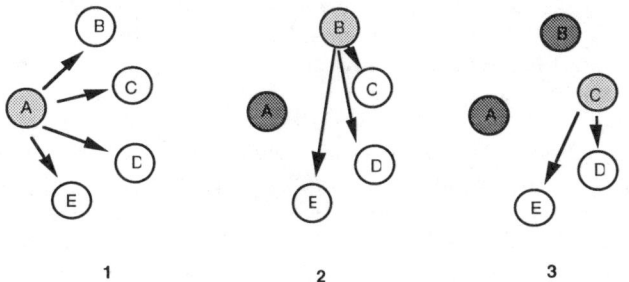

Fig. 13.1 *Three generations of exposures and transmissions of an infection in a family with five children. White denotes susceptible, grey infectious, and black immune. Arrows denote exposures.*

A exposes four susceptibles, and then becomes immune. In the second generation, B exposes three susceptibles, and in the third, C only exposes two susceptibles, since A and B are already immune. In this example there would thus be nine exposures of susceptibles total.

This method of counting every new round of exposures due to the secondary, tertiary, etc. cases in the family gives a figure for the attack rate that Hope Simpson calls the 'susceptible exposure attack rate'. It is a very well-defined measure of infectivity, but sometimes quite difficult to attain. An alternative measure is called 'household secondary attack rate' where all nonprimary cases in a household are lumped together in the calculation. In the example above, the household AR would be 50%, since two out of four siblings were infected. The susceptible exposure AR according to Hope Simpson would only be 2/9, or 22%. You see that it becomes crucial exactly how one defines the measure of attack rate. In order to calculate susceptible exposure attack rate, it is also very important to sort out the generations of cases.

For both types of measures of AR, there may be a problem with the true number of susceptibles: whereas subclinical cases of measles are rare, chickenpox can sometimes be very discrete, and a mumps infection can be quite asymptomatic. Some children may thus have been regarded as susceptible who were in fact immune. The figure we are looking for is the number of transmissions divided by the number of susceptible children exposed, but if exposures of immune children are entered into the denominator, then the attack rate calculated will be too low. The problem will be worse for the susceptible exposure attack rate method, since counting such exposures twice will increase the magnitude of this error.

Another problem concerns how multiple exposures should be accounted for. If there are two simultaneous primary cases in the household, how many exposures do the siblings receive?

Hope Simpson carefully underlines that his estimates of attack rates only apply to spread within families, and that other studies must be performed to assess attack rates in other settings. It might be added that the figures only strictly apply to families of the sizes and living conditions that were prevalent in western England around 1950.

A rather similar study of household attack rates was performed in the USA in the late 70s.[2] The issue was to measure the risk of household spread of invasive *Haemophilus influenzae* (HI) infections.

The index cases were patients with HI meningitis reported to the state health departments in 20 American states during an 18-month period. One thousand four hundred and three such patients had their infections confirmed by culture of blood or cerebrospinal fluid. The families of 1,147 of these patients were then investigated by the state or local health department, who assessed the number of actual contacts in each household and followed them for 30 days after the index case fell ill. Secondary household cases were again confirmed by isolation of HI from blood or CSF. In total, there were 4,311 household contacts, of whom 1,687 were less than six years of age.

This study is also an example of a cohort design, in which all exposed family members are followed to assess the risk of infection. The study might have been prospective: if index cases were reported quickly, and the health department visited the families immediately, or retrospective: if there was a delay in reporting, and the 30 days had already passed when the health department came around. It is also an example of passive surveillance to find the index cases, and of active surveillance to find the secondary cases.

Nine associated cases of serious HI infection in eight households occurred within 30 days after onset of meningitis in the index case. The risk of transmission was calculated by age of the susceptibles (Table 13.1).

Table 13.1 *Household attack rate of* Haemophilus influenza *infection by age in a study from the USA.* Source: *Ward* et al.[2]

Age	No. at risk	No. ill	Risk (%)	95% confidence interval
<1 year	50	3	6.0	1.3–16.6
1 year	69	1	1.4	0.04–7.8
2–3 years	259	4	1.5	0.4–4.0
4–5 years	1309	1	0.1	0.002–0.4
6–9 years	607	0	0	0–0.6
10–19 years	431	0	0	0–0.9
≥20 years	1586	0	0	0–0.2
Total	4311	9	0.21	0.10–0.40

The confidence intervals were calculated with the method for proportions described in Chapter 6. One can see that there was a marked difference in attack rates depending on age, with no cases appearing in contacts six years or older. This means that age would be an important confounder if one were to compare attack rate of HI meningitis in two different populations.

Seventy percent of the associated cases occurred within one week of the index patient's disease, and the median serial interval for this type of infection should thus be less than a week. The incubation period might be longer, if the primary cases were infectious for some time before they fell ill.

This study gives a low estimate for the attack rate of serious HI infection, since index cases as well as contacts had to have a severe, laboratory-proven infection. Other forms of HI disease, such as pneumonia, cellulitis or otitis media might add to the risk of illness in household contacts, but they were not included. Since there was one family with two secondary cases (or one secondary and one tertiary), the authors might have used the Hope Simpson definition of secondary attack rate in this household, but they only give the crude rates of the table above.

The authors also made use of serotyping to show that all the invasive infections in index and secondary cases were caused by HI type b, which is known to be more virulent than other HI strains.

This possibility of 'finger-printing' the infectious agent is a nice feature of infectious disease epidemiology. If one thinks about it, it is really a continuous process that started with the discovery of bacteria in the last century. It would for example be very difficult to study the epidemiology of diarrhoea without the tools to single out the different species that cause this condition. The next step was the advent of serology some 60 years ago, which taught us to differentiate within species, thus adding to the possibility of following the path of a pathogen through the population. A good example is given by the subtyping of *Salmonella* species, which can help us to discover outbreaks and eliminate a source even if the overall incidence of salmonella infections is almost constant, just as was exemplified by the chocolate bar outbreak in the previous chapter. The present leap are the different methods for 'genetic fingerprinting', which allow us to identify individual strains of bacteria or viruses by looking at specific sequences in their genomes. With methods such as 'restriction-fragment length polymorphism', it is often possible to chart the separate chains of infection within a population where several sources of the same pathogen are operating simultaneously.

Other examples – sexually transmitted infections

The sexual transmission of infections provides another field of study, where the type of contact is sufficiently standardized to allow for calculations of attack rates. As part of the previously cited study on chlamydia infection in Sweden, data from partner notification was utilized to calculate the risk of transmission of this bacteria.[3]

Almost 6,000 young women were screened for chlamydia infection in a number of family planning clinics in Gothenburg. None of them had subjective symptoms of a genital infection, but 425 were found to be culture positive for chlamydia. For 309 of these women it was possible to contact and test the male partner with whom they had last had intercourse before the diagnosis was made. Seventy-four of these men, or 24%, also had a chlamydia infection.

At first sight this looks like another nice cohort study, where 309 men were exposed to 309 women with chlamydia infection. We know that the women could not have become infected later, since this was their last intercourse before diagnosis. The attack rate of chlamydia infection would then be 24%. However, there are several difficulties involved in the interpretation of data like these: firstly, we do not know who infected whom. Some of the infected men must have been the sources of the infections in the women, and were thus neither exposed nor susceptible. Secondly, some of the men could have been infected by another partner after their intercourse with an index woman. Thirdly, the median time between diagnosis of the index case and testing of the partner was 21 days, and for 10% of the men it was more than two months. Several men might have recovered from their infections – or had perhaps been taking antibiotics for other infections that cured their chlamydia infection as well. Fourthly, even if the figure 24% were correct, it need not apply to the risk of transmission from an infected male to a susceptible female.

Studies of the attack rate of STDs thus have several methodological problems, and many published studies are more like case reports where it has been possible to calculate the number of transmissions to partners of one single infectious individual.

As a rare example of the opposite, a rather elegant study on the risk of gonorrhoea transmission from females to males was made in the early 1970s on the crew members of a large US Navy vessel.[4] During the passage across the Pacific Ocean, all sailors were tested for gonorrhoea infection, and the ones found to be infected were treated. The ship subsequently spent four days in an Asian port, during which time the crew had the opportunity to meet local prostitutes and barmaids. After leaving port, a sample of 537 men were again examined for gonorrhoea infection, and 54 were now positive. The overall attack rate was thus 10%, but that figure tells us nothing about transmission risk unless we also know prevalence on infection in the women. This important piece of extra information was provided from the clinic that the registered prostitutes had to attend for bimonthly check-ups. Five hundred and eleven out of the approximately 8,000 prostitutes in the area attended this clinic during the days when the ship was in port, and they were all examined for gonorrhoea. Ninety of them were infected, for a prevalence of 17.6%.

The next step in the calculations requires two assumptions: the first is that the 511 women examined constituted a representative sample of all the women that the crew could have met. The second is that the men chose women randomly as regards infectious status: the women who were infected should not have higher or lower probability of becoming a partner than the ones who were not infected. If these two assumptions hold, then 17.6% of the men would have been exposed to gonorrhoea, and since 10% became infected, risk of transmission (= attack rate) would be 10/17.6 = 57%.

Many models for the spread of STDs assume a constant attack rate per intercourse, and that the risk of transmission will increase with the number of intercourses that an infectious and a susceptible have. This is a good place to introduce a parenthesis about the calculation of risk in such situations. Let us assume that we are studying an STD for which there is some empirical evidence that the attack rate after one act of intercourse is 25%. For someone who was unfamiliar with statistics it could be easy to believe that the risk of becoming infected after four acts of intercourse with an infectious partner would be $4 \times 25 = 100\%$, but that is wrong. Risks cannot be added like that, and the problem is somewhat similar to the discussion of risks and rates in Chapter 9. The reason for this is that the way of becoming infected in, say, the third intercourse is to escape infection in the first two, and then being infected in the third. The probability of this event is lower than 25%. The simplest way to estimate the total risk is as follows: first calculate the probability of *not* being infected at all during the four intercourses. This is equal to the chance of escaping infection the first time, which is 75%, multiplied by the chance of not being infected the second time, which is again 75%, and so on. The probability of not being infected after four acts of intercourse is thus $0.75 \times 0.75 \times 0.75 \times 0.75 = 0.32$. Next remember that the probability of something happening is 1 minus the probability that it does not happen, which means that the risk of *having* become infected is $1 - 0.32$, or 0.68. The risk is thus 68% after four acts of intercourse, and not 100%. End of parenthesis.

In the example of gonorrhoea among the naval crew above, the authors tried to use this formula to calculate the risk per act of sexual intercourse, since most of the men had had intercourse more than once with each partner. They arrive at the unexplained finding that the attack rate per intercourse in the white sailors was 19%, but as high as 53% in black crew members. They discuss that one possible reason for this could be a selection bias among the women, in that the prostitutes that the white men met might have had a lower gonorrhoea prevalence.

We will be looking at more studies that measure attack rate in the chapter on vaccines later in the book.

Dose

Another important aspect of infectivity concerns the dose of the pathogen that a susceptible person receives. You should observe that there is a close connection between the concept of 'dose' and the concept 'type of contact' discussed previously: a closer contact between an infectious and a susceptible will probably lead to the transmission of a higher dose.

In most real-life situations it becomes almost impossible to measure the infective dose, counted as number of bacteria or viruses. How do we know exactly how many virus particles a measles case spreads when coughing? How many of these must enter a susceptible individual to cause infection and/or disease? We know that the blood of an acute case of hepatitis B may contain up to 10^9 virus particles per ml, but in the study of percutaneous, accidental transmission in the hospital, how do we know the exact volume of blood inoculated into a susceptible person?

For enteric infections, the relationship between dose and risk of infection has been studied quite well in regular trials. Several such trials took place in the US in the 1950s and 1960s, and used prisoner volunteers as subjects.

In one such experiment,[5] controlled doses of *Salmonella bareilly* were given to three groups of six volunteers. Table 13.2 shows the results.

Table 13.2 *Attack rate as a function of ingested dose of bacteria.* Source: *McCollough and Eisle[5]*

Dose	Ill	Well	AR (%)
125,000	1	5	17
695,000	2	4	33
1,700,000	4	2	67

The attack rate clearly increases with dose, and it seems that a dose of around 1,000,000 bacteria will cause disease in half the subjects exposed. This figure is sometimes called ID_{50} (= the dose of a pathogen that will cause disease in 50% of exposed susceptibles). A possible error in calculations such as these is that some of the ill subjects were not infected in the experiment, but that they became secondary cases to some real primary case. The authors assure the reader, however, that this could not have happened. One should also note that the number involved in the study was small and therefore the confidence intervals for the attack rates will be very wide (for the estimate 33% in the middle line in the table the 95% confidence interval will be from −5 to 71%, using the formula for a proportion in Chapter 6).

In this definition of attack rate, only clinical cases were counted. Changes in agglutination titres (a serological, rather crude test for salmonella infection) were also measured in all subjects, but only showed any rise in four of the seven cases. However, the number of days that the subjects excreted *Salmonella* in faeces are shown in Fig. 13.2 below.

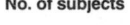

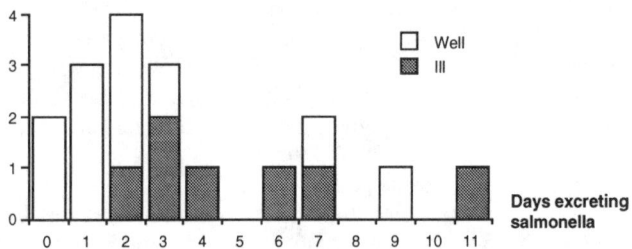

Fig. 13.2 *Number of days salmonella could be found in stools in 18 volunteers given controlled doses of* Salmonella bareilly .
Source: *McCollough and Eisele*[5]

That is: two of the subjects only excreted *Salmonella* on the day of the trial, three of them continued to excrete *Salmonella* during the next day, but not longer, and so on. Most of the subjects who did not fall ill thus excreted the bacteria for a day or two only, which may have been just those bacteria they had ingested. However, the two well subjects who excreted *Salmonella* for seven and nine days probably had subclinical infections. They were both given the medium dose.

This example once again shows the importance of the case definition in calculating attack rates. When reading studies on ARs or on infectivity, one should always check if subclinical cases were included or not, and how they were ascertained.

In a similar study of typhoid,[6] volunteers were given controlled doses of *Salmonella typhii* with a 10^6 variation in number of bacteria given (Table 13.3).

Table 13.3 *Attack rate of* Salmonella typhii *infection with increasing doses of bacteria ingested.*   Source: *Hornick* et al.[6]

Dose	Ill	Well	AR (%)
10^3	0	14	0
10^5	32	84	28
10^7	16	16	50
10^8	8	1	89
10^9	40	2	95

In this example also, the ID_{50} seems to be around 1,000,000 bacteria, and the higher number of subjects in each group give better confidence intervals for the ARs than in the previous example.

In some outbreaks, it has been possible to get an estimate of infective dose in 'real life' situations. For bacterial enteric infections this becomes possible if some part of the infected food item remains and can be tested after the outbreak has been discovered. One example comes from an outbreak of *Salmonella eastbourne* in North America in 1974[7].

The outbreak was spread over several states in the US and in Canada. It was discovered by the US national surveillance programme. Shortly after the detection of the outbreak, a telephone-based case-control study was undertaken, interviewing 28 cases in different states. Only primary cases in each family were interviewed, and each family was asked to name two controls. The odds ratio for having eaten a certain brand of Christmas-wrapped chocolate balls was 9 with a narrow confidence interval. Several families still had chocolate balls at home, and samples for salmonella infection were taken from them. The mean number of bacteria was 2.5 per gram. The investigators assumed that a typical case would have eaten 1 lb. of chocolate, for a total dose of 1,000 bacteria, much lower than in the experiment above.

Several other studies have shown lower doses in outbreaks from food or water than in the controlled experiments above. There is obviously always a problem to know that the density of bacteria remaining some days to weeks after the exposure is the same as it was originally. This can sometimes be assessed by controlled contamination of similar food, which is then subjected to the same process (freezing, etc.) as the source of the outbreak. However, chocolate is a particularly good medium in this respect, since *Salmonella* bacteria are stable in chocolate.

Numerical calculations of infective doses can thus sometimes be made for enteric infections, where the number of infecting organisms can be measured or estimated. For most other infections, and especially for those that are spread by contact or via the air, this is generally impossible. In estimating the relationship between dose and attack rate for such infections one will thus have to use closeness of contact as a proxy measure for dose, assuming that a susceptible who is near a case for a long time will be exposed to a higher dose than a casual contact of the same case.

We have already seen one example of different attack rates for different types of contacts in the example of monkeypox in Chapter 3. A similar study was made during an outbreak of smallpox in a village in Dahomey in 1967[8].

The disease was introduced into the village with some 300 inhabitants by a woman and her two children, who all developed smallpox around the time of their arrival. It spread to eight other houses during two and a half months. Six of these houses were immediate neighbours.

The household attack rate in the nine afflicted houses was 17 cases out of 34 exposed, or 50%. The number of transmissions to someone outside the household was 7, and based on denominator of around 270 (since 34 of all the people in the village were household contacts), the attack rate between households would be some 3%. This indicates that close and prolonged contact is usually necessary for spread, and it is difficult to think of any explanation for this other than a correlation between risk of infection and dose.

Immunity

This problem was touched on above concerning the Hope Simpson data. Immune persons should not be entered among the susceptibles exposed. It is often not possible to know whether a person was immune when exposed, and even if a serology could be performed after the exposure, one may not always be able to tell a previous immunity from a subclinical infection due to the exposure.

One nice example of the opposite comes from a measles outbreak in a dormitory at a US university in 1985[9].

Between 31 January and 7 February the Red Cross held a blood drive at the university, asking the students to donate blood. Almost simultaneously, a measles outbreak started there, the first case being diagnosed 28 January, and the last 20 March. A lot of the students would thus have had blood samples taken just before the outbreak started. One hundred and thirty-nine students living in the dormitory had donated blood, and 90 of these agreed to take part in a study, the aim of which was to analyse the association between antibody titres before exposure and subsequent risk of measles.

A measles case was defined as an illness characterized by generalized maculopapular rash of more than three days duration, fever greater than $38.3^{\circ}C$ if measured, and at least one of the following: cough, coryza or conjunctivitis. They were confirmed by blood samples showing a four-fold or higher rise in antibody titre from the acute to the convalescent sample (see Chapter 15 for a discussion of antibody titres). One student developed a rash just three days after donating blood, and was excluded, since his antibody titre at the time of donation might already have been on the rise.

Donated blood is usually kept in plastic bags, but there is always some blood left in the plastic tube leading into the bag (the 'pigtail'), and this blood could be collected for 80 of the 90 subjects of the study. Eight of the 90 donors had an illness meeting the clinical case definition, and measles was confirmed serologically in seven of these (post-illness sera were unavailable for 1). If a pre-exposure antibody titre value of 1/120 was chosen of cut-off, the outcome was a follows:

	Antibody titre ≤ 1/120	Antibody titre > 1/120	
Measles	8	0	8
No measles	1	71	72
	9	71	80

The difference is highly significant ($p < 0.001$ by Fisher's exact test), and we can see that just one person with a low titre escaped infection. This is thus a very nice example of how immunity influences attack rate in an outbreak.

It is difficult to think of any biases or confounders that could have distorted this finding. The students who volunteered for the study hardly had any knowledge of their pre-exposure titres, and all blood tests were made blind of the case status of the student. One possibility would be that the antibody measured had nothing to do with protection, but rather was a marker for some real protective factor, but then the correlation between this confounder and the real factor must have been very high. The investigators could also show a raise in antibody titre in a number of students who did not develop measles, and we will return to those results in a later chapter.

Other cofactors

This chapter makes no attempt to list all the factors that influence risk of infection. One often mentioned example is the increased risk of enteric infections, and especially cholera, in patients who suffer from achlorhydria of the stomach. The very low pH of the ventricle is an important defence mechanism against several infections.

We will just look at a somewhat unusual study that tried to relate the degree of psychological stress to infection rate from common cold viruses.[10]

The study was performed at the Medical Research Council's Common Cold Unit in Salisbury – an institution that has produced several interesting results on the epidemiology of common colds. The subjects were 154 men and 266 women volunteers, aged 18 to 54. During the first two days the subjects underwent a thorough medical examination, and answered three different questionnaires designed to measure their present degree of psychological stress. Subsequently, a solution containing either one of five different viruses or saline placebo was dropped into each subject's nose, and they were then put in quarantine and monitored for infection and clinical symptoms.

The occurrence of infection was established with both virological and serological criteria. Clinical cold was established by subjects' reports and by clinical examination.

The results were analysed by logistic regression, where the outcome measure was either laboratory verified infection or clinical cold. The explanatory factor was the degree of psychological stress as scored by the questionnaires. For both outcomes there was a significant increase in attack rate with increasing stress score: the rate of infection ranged from 74–90% and the incidence of clinical cold from 27–47% going from lowest to highest stress value. These findings remained significant even after controlling for a number of confounders such as age, allergic status, season, and virus-specific antibody status at baseline. Simply dividing the subjects into those with high versus those with low stress gave an adjusted OR for infection of 5.8 and for illness of 2.2. The associations were similar for all five strains of virus tested. This study probably supports the popular belief that one becomes more susceptible to infection when feeling stressed.

Subclinical infections

As I have mentioned in several places now, the value for an attack rate very much depends on how a 'case' is defined. In many studies, the numerator only includes the cases that were diagnosed clinically. However, most people would probably want to include subclinical infections as well, especially if those patients can spread the disease further in the population. If such cases are to be detected, one needs serology, and in some instances one needs a sample taken before the exposure for comparison. This happened to be the case in the example above, but is generally a quite rare event.

Parenthetically, it should be noted that measles is one of the best diseases available for studying transmission, which has always made it a favourite with infectious disease epidemiologists: attack rate is high, there are very few subclinical cases, the incubation time is short, and immunity after infection is lifelong in most cases. There are not many other infections for which these four statements are true, and taking HIV infection as an example, the opposite of each statement applies.

Summary

Infectivity must be distinguished from 'risk of becoming infected', since this risk will also depend on prevalence of infectious sources in the environment (mosquitoes, people, etc.).

It is not clear why not all susceptible become infected when exposed. Dose of the pathogen is one important factor, but even with identical doses some people are infected and others not. Perhaps there exist temporary fluctuations in some kind of nonspecific immunological resistance, but such would be very difficult to study. In the absence of exact biological understanding of the factors governing infection in every single case, we resort to talking about the probability, or risk, of disease after a certain kind of exposure. This measure we call the attack rate.

The relationship between attack rate and dose can be studied in cohort studies, both by ingestion of a known number of bacteria and in natural situations, where dose ingested can be estimated afterwards. For diseases that are spread person-to-person, closeness and duration of contact between an infectious and a susceptible individual is often taken as a proxy measure of dose transmitted.

When measuring attack rates for diseases that are spread from person to person, careful elucidation of transmission routes and generations is essential. There exist several definitions of attack rate in such situations, and the susceptible exposure attack rate is probably the best defined and the one which best measures infectivity. It is, however, very sensitive to the erroneous inclusion of already immune subjects as exposed susceptibles.

References

1. Hope Simpson RE. Infectiousness of communicable diseases in the household (measles, chickenpox and mumps). *Lancet* 1952; **2**: 549–54.

2. Ward JI, Fraser DW, Baraff LJ, Plikaytis BD. *Hemophilus influenzae* meningitis. A national study of secondary spread in household contacts. *N Engl J Med* 1979: **301**: 122–26.

3. Ramstedt K, Forssman L, Giesecke J, Johannisson G. Epidemiological characteristics of two different populations of women with *Chlamydia trachomatis* infection and their male partners. *Sex Transm Dis* 1991; **18**: 46–51.

4. Hooper RR, Reynolds GH, Jones OG, *et al.* Cohort study of venereal disease. I: The risk of gonorrhea transmission from infected women to men. *Am J Epidemiol* 1978; **108**: 136–45.

5. McCullough NB, Eisele CW. Experimental human salmonellosis. III. Pathogenicity of strains of *Salmonella newport*, *Salmonella derby*, and *Salmomella bareilly* obtained from spray-dried whole egg. *J Infect Dis* 1951; **89**: 209–13.

6. Hornick RB, Greisman SE, Woodward TE, DuPont HL, Dawkins AT, Snyder MJ. Typhoid fever: Pathogenesis and immunologic control. *N Engl J Med* 1970; **283**: 686–91.

7. Craven PC, Baine WB, Mackel DC, *et al.* International outbreak of *Salmonella eastbourne* infection traced to contaminated chocolate. *Lancet* 1975; **1**: 788–92.

8. Henderson RH, Yekpe M. Smallpox transmission in Southern Dahomey. A study of a village outbreak. *Am J Epidemiol* 1969; **90**: 423–28.

9. Chen RT, Markowitz LE, Albrecht P, *et al.* Measles antibody: reevaluation of protective titers. *J Infect Dis* 1990; **162**: 1036–42.

10.Cohen S, Tyrell DAJ, Smith AP. Psychological stress and the susceptibility to common cold. *N Eng J Med* 1991: **325**: 606–12.

14 Studying the natural history of infectious diseases

Here the epidemiological methods to study the natural history of an infectious disease are touched upon, as well as the study of prognostic markers and co-factors for disease progression. Biases in such studies are discussed, and the importance of dose is once again exemplified.

This book deals more with the transmission, detection, diagnosis and prevention of infectious diseases than with their natural history and treatment. The reason for this is that the first four points are more particular to infectious disease epidemiology; once a patient has become a case and starts developing the disease or is taken into hospital the tools used for epidemiological study become similar for almost all groups of diseases.

Important questions concerning the natural history of an infectious disease are: what is the incubation time? what are the symptoms? how severe is the disease generally, and what are the risk factors for a more serious course of events? how long does the infection last? We have already encountered one such concept in Chapter 2: the case fatality rate, which measures how many of those who acquire an infection will die from in within some defined time period.

A very much related question concerns the effects of different drugs such as antibiotics and antivirals on the severity and outcome of a disease. Such questions are generally studied in regular clinical trials, with randomization, controlling and blinding. You will remember from Chapter 5 that the main conceptual difference between 'pure' epidemiological studies and clinical trials, is that for the former we have to be content with the assignment of risk factors and subjects that nature provides, whereas for the latter we can choose subjects and assign exposures at will.

Incubation periods

The easiest way to measure an incubation period is obviously in an outbreak situation, when a group of people were exposed simultaneously. The epidemic curve of such an outbreak will give a good picture of the incubation time distribution, and if you remember the Legionnaire's disease outbreak in Chapter 11 you may recall that the incubation time for this new disease was actually known before the aetiology was clarified. In more prolonged outbreaks, or when the infection is transmitted from person to person, one will need to interview cases carefully about when they could have been exposed.

One of the nicest such studies performed is also one of the oldest. It comes from an outbreak of measles in the Faroe Islands, west of the coast of Norway in 1846. At that time, these islands were part of Denmark, and the young doctor Panum was sent by the authorities to investigate the outbreak.[1] In the report on the investigation, he points out that:

'... The isolated situation of the villages, and their limited intercourse with each other, made it possible in many, in fact in most, cases to ascertain where and when the person who first fell ill had been exposed to the infection, and to prove that the contagion could not have affected him either before or after the day stated. ...'

He interviewed a large number of cases, and seems to have followed the infection in almost every village of the islands, clarifying exactly who brought the infection to the village, and where he or she must have been infected. The clearest example relates to the village of Tjörnevig. On the 4th of June a boat with 10 men from Tjörnevig had gone to the village of Vestmannhavn to take part in a hunt for grind (a small whale). They spent some time in houses there, and Panum could later record that there had been measles cases in these houses during the days subsequent to the visit. On June 18th, exactly 14 days after the exposure, measles rash broke out in every one of the 10 men, after they had been feeling ill with cough and conjunctivitis for two to four days. Almost everyone else in Tjörnevig then developed a measles rash between 12 and 16 days later, except for a few who fell ill some 12 to 16 days after the first general outbreak.

From similar observations in other villages, Panum drew the conclusion that the incubation time from exposure to first symptoms of measles was 10 to 12 days, and to rash 14 days. The shortest serial interval was 12 days, showing that a case was infectious some two days before the rash developed.

He also made another observation concerning the natural history of measles, namely that case fatality rate (CFR) increased with age. By comparing with average mortality from parish registers for the time period 1835 to 1845 he could show that during the period of the epidemic, overall mortality did not change at all in the age group one to 20 years, whilst in the age group 30–50 it increased by a factor of 2.5, and for the 50-60 year olds by a factor of 5.

Another finding, which has few parallels in infectious disease epidemiology, was factual data to support that measles infection confers life-long immunity. The previous measles epidemic on the Faroes had been in 1781, 65 years earlier, and since then the disease had been totally absent from the islands. Panum observed that not one single person who had had measles in 1781 and who was still alive in 1846 had the disease a second time.

Natural history

The basic type of design for studying the natural history of an infectious disease is the cohort study. A cohort of patients that have been diagnosed with the disease are followed over time, and events and outcomes recorded. In many such studies, a bias regarding severity is introduced, which may or may not be a problem depending on point of view. Since they are generally based on patients diagnosed within the health-care system, and often on patients in hospital, they will tend to include patients whose disease is towards the more severe end of a scale. Asymptomatic or mild infections will not be diagnosed or included.

For several important diseases, the ratio of subclinical to clinical infections in an epidemic is very high. It has been estimated that for every apparent child with polio in an epidemic there are about 100 asymptomatic infected children in the population. Cholera is another disease where many become infected but few fall ill. In the absence of serology or bacterial culture, the normal natural history of such infections will not be properly understood.

If the results of a study on hospitalized patients are used to describe the natural history of a disease, the prognosis will seem worse than a general practitioner would find from his experiences, and even worse than a study that was based on all cases in the population. An infectious disease doctor may find that quite a high proportion of salmonella patients develop complications to the infection, such as arthritis or arteritis. However, since only a small proportion of salmonella infections are diagnosed, and an ever smaller proportion are seen in the hospital, the overall risk may not be very high.

On the other hand, if the aim of the study is not to describe the general natural history, but rather to inform hospital doctors about the complications they are likely to see, then such a study would not be biased – provided that the selection of patients is similar in the clinics where the study is read.

One example of a study that gives preliminary information on the natural history of a newly discovered disease comes from Venezuela[2]: in September 1989, an outbreak of a severe haemorrhagic disease was observed by physicians in Guanarito. It was first believed to be dengue, but one year later a new virus was isolated from a fatal case, and a serological test for this new Guanarito virus was developed from mouse ascitic fluid. From September 1990 through April 1991, 14 patients treated in a hospital in Guanare were diagnosed to be infected with this virus, either by isolation or by seroconversion.

The age range of the patients was from six to 54 years, with most of the cases in young adults, and they had been ill between three and 12 days before admission. The main presenting symptoms were fever, prostration, arthralgia and headache, and 13 of the 14 patients had one or more haemorrhagic manifestations. Nine of the 14 patients died within one to six days after admission.

The case fatality rate in this study was $9/14 = 0.64$, but the sample is small. Let us use our formula for confidence interval for a proportion from Chapter 6 to calculate a 95% confidence interval. The standard error of this proportion will be:

$$\sqrt{\frac{0.64 \times 0.36}{14}} = 0.128$$

and the 95% confidence interval is given by $0.64 \pm 2 \times 0.128$, which means that the CFR for this disease would be between 38% and 90%. The confidence interval becomes wide when the sample is small.

A more serious objection to the figure for the CFR concerns the selection of subjects. The authors remark that their case fatality rate is higher than reported for Lassa fever or Argentinean haemorrhagic fever, but also that early studies on these diseases found very high rates, which have later been modified when milder cases are diagnosed. They thus undertook a small seroepidemiological study of 57 family contacts of the cases and found six of those to have antibody to Guanarito virus, which supports the notion that the patients seen in the hospital represented a more severe form of the disease.

Prognostic factors

Similar cohort strategies can also be used to study factors in individual patients with a certain disease that will be associated with outcome. An example of the basic structure of such studies is given by an investigation of the association between size of vegetation and outcome in infectious endocarditis in the USA.[3]

The study focused on right-sided endocarditis in intravenous drug users. It was performed as a retrospective cohort study, in which the medical records of 121 such patients with 132 episodes of active endocarditis were reviewed. They had been treated in the Beth Israel Medical Center once or more during the years 1978 to 1986, and the inclusion criteria were: right-sided valvular vegetation documented by two-dimensional echocardiography, history of intravenous drug use, two or more positive blood cultures, and at least two clinical signs compatible with active endocarditis (fever, septic emboli, heart murmur).

The authors used only two endpoints: death or discharge without any clinical signs of active endocarditis. In 30 of the 132 episodes, the patients left the hospital before completion of treatment, and these were not included in the analysis. Of the remaining 102 episodes, 10 ended with the patient's death, and 92 were successfully treated. Three of the patients who died had complications other than a right-sided vegetation, and one of the cured patients had a prosthetic valve. These four patients were excluded from the analysis of native valve vegetation size and outcome (Table 14.1).

Table 14.1 *Mortality as a function of valvular vegetation size in a study on right-sided endocarditis.*   Source: *Hecht and Berger*[2]

Vegetation size	No. of episodes	Mortality (%)
≤ 1 cm	19	0
1.1 – 2 cm	61	2
> 2 cm	18	33

Evidently, the risk of dying increases with increasing size of the vegetation, and the difference in risk between the last group and the first two combined is highly significant.

The authors also analysed if prolonged fever, lasting more than three weeks, had any adverse effect on outcome, but did not find any such association.

This study is also instructive because it underlines the difficulties in performing epidemiological studies in the clinic, even under the best of circumstances. From the original intended 132 episodes to be analysed, 34 had to be excluded for different reasons: a dropout rate that I would describe as quite normal. One could speculate how the 30 episodes when the patient left the hospital too early would have influenced the result. The article does not tell how long they stayed in the hospital, but the median number of treatment days for those who died was around 10. It might be assumed that those who left had less severe disease, and that their inclusion would decrease the overall CFR, but in the absence of any data on those patients this must remain a guess.

Dose and severity of disease

An important issue in the discussion of natural history of infectious diseases is whether a higher dose at infection leads to a more severe disease. Since most pathogens divide and multiply at a high rate, it is not self-evident that the actual number received is of any significance; the number will increase rapidly anyway. In the example with the volunteers ingesting *Salmonella typhii* in Chapter 13, there did not seem to be any such correlation, even if the average incubation period was shorter with higher dose.

The relationship between dose, measured as amount of contact between case and susceptible and severity of measles infection was studied in an area in Senegal.[4]

The foundation for the study was a surveillance system operating in 30 villages with a total population around 24,000. The villages were made up of compounds, where on average 14 people lived, although some could have over 100 inhabitants. Within each compound there were a number of households (of average size eight), defined as a group of people who normally ate together, and each household in turn occupied a number of huts (average 2.5 persons per hut). Measles cases in children were reported by their parents, and clinically confirmed by a physician. No serological samples were taken. Cases not seen by a physician were still included if they were linked epidemiologically to other known cases in the same compound or the same village.

The investigators wanted to study the case fatality rate for measles in this population. One then has to decide how late after the disease death could occur, and still be regarded as due to the infection. In studies on measles, deaths up to six weeks after the appearance of rash are usually attributed to the infection, and this limit was chosen here also.

Between 1983 and 1986, 1,500 cases of measles were reported and 98 of these died within six weeks for an overall CFR of 6.5%. The CFR varied quite widely with age, from over 10% for children aged between six months and three years to 0% in children over 10 and in adults. Simply dividing the cases into those younger or older than 41 months (3.5 years) at onset gives us the CFR shown in Table 14.2.

Table 14.2   *Case fatality rate (CFR) in measles by age in an area of Senegal*   Source: *Garenne and Aaby.*[4]

Age, months	Cases	Deaths	CFR (%)
4 – 41	735	87	12
≥ 42	765	11	1.4

The first case diagnosed in a compound was regarded as primary, and cases appearing in the same compound 6 – 16 days after the primary case were called secondary. – Of course, there is always some uncertainty about the actual source of the secondary cases, they could also have become infected outside the compound, but if the onset of disease fell within the right serial interval, they were still counted as secondary. If there were several simultaneous primary cases in a compound, the source of exposure for each secondary case was assumed to be the closest one, i.e. in the same hut, same household, or same compound, in that order. One appreciates how meticulously time of onset and location of each case must be collected in a study like this.

For 190 cases there was no adequate information on exposure. Of the remaining, 402 were classified as primary and 908 as secondary. For each of the secondary cases the type of exposure to its primary case was assessed. The CFRs according to type of exposure are given in Table 14.3.

If we set the risk of dying = 1 if a child was exposed in the compound only, then the relative risks for the secondary cases become

7.1/5.4 = 1.31 for exposure in a household, and 9.9/5.4 = 1.83 for in-hut exposure. These differences are significant, and point to that closeness of contact affects severity of disease, measured as fatality.

Table 14.3 *Same study as in Table 14.2, now showing case fatality rate (CFR) in secondary cases depending on place of exposure.*

Exposure	Cases	Deaths	CFR (%)
Secondary in:			
Compound	203	11	5.4
Household	310	22	7.1
Hut	395	39	9.9

However, let us use this nice study for a recapitulation of confounders and how to control for them. The next to last table showed that age was strongly inversely associated with risk of dying. If we divide the secondary cases according to how they were exposed, it seems likely for example that infants would be more likely to be exposed in a hut than running around in the compound. We thus have every reason to believe that place of exposure would also be associated with age, and that age of the secondary case could be a confounder.

We thus re-tabulate the secondary cases, this time making two tables, one for children aged 41 months or less (Table 14.4) and one for those aged 42 months or more (Table 14.5).

Table 14.4 *Case fatality rate (CFR) in secondary cases aged 4 to 41 months. RR relative risk.*

Exposure	Cases	Deaths	CFR (%)	RR (compound = 1)
Secondary in:				
Compound	91	10	11.0	1
Household	158	18	11.4	1.04
Hut	189	33	17.5	1.59

Table 14.5 *Case fatality rate (CFR) in secondary cases aged 42 months or more. RR relative risk.*

Exposure	Cases	Deaths	CFR (%)	RR (compound = 1)
Secondary in:				
Compound	112	1	0.9	1
Household	152	4	2.6	2.89
Hut	206	6	2.9	3.22

The effect of exposure thus seems even more pronounced in the older children. (One should observe, however, that only one case infected in the compound died in the older group, and that the calculation of RRs is quite uncertain; confidence intervals would be wide.)

If one wants to avoid having two tables, and just give one age-adjusted RR for the each type of contact, one uses the Mantel-Haenszel (MH) method described in Chapter 8. The cases exposed in the compound would be the base-line group, and we would have two age groups for exposure in the household and two for in-hut exposure. For the two groups exposed in the household, the MH weight for the younger children would be:

$$w_{4-41} = 10 \times 158/(91 + 158) = 6.34$$

which is read as 'for the children in the younger group, the weight is calculated as the number of deaths in the baseline group (10) multiplied by all cases in the household group (158) divided by the sum of cases in the two groups (91 + 158)'.

For children in the older group, the weight becomes:

$$w_{42-} = 1 \times 152/(112 + 152) = 0.58$$

We see that the weight for the RR in the older group is much lower, due to the fact that there was only one case in the baseline (=compound) group.

Each weight is multiplied with its corresponding RR and the overall RR for dying after exposure in the household compared to the risk of dying after exposure in the compound regardless of age becomes

$$RR_{MH} = \frac{1.04 \times 6.34 + 2.89 \times 0.58}{6.34 + 0.58} = 1.20$$

which is clearly lower than the crude RR given under the first table, which was 1.31. In similar fashion, the RR_{MH} for dying after exposure in the hut is calculated as 1.73, which is also lower than the crude relative risk of 1.83. In this example, exposure was thus confounded by age, in that the children who had the closest exposure also tended to be the younger children.

This study shows a clear relationship between dose and severity. It was performed as a cohort study, where all cases of measles were followed up. An alternative approach would have been to make a case-control study, where the children who died would have been the cases, and a sample of the surviving cases could be taken a controls (the terminology gets a bit muddled in a situation like this). The pattern of exposure could then have been compared in the two groups.

Other cofactors for severity

The list of cofactors that influence the course of an infection once it has been established is very long. This book only looks at a few of these, the reasons being, firstly, that they are usually studied with research methods already described here and which are not unique to infectious disease epidemiology and, secondly, that they really belong more in a textbook on infectious disease medicine. The two examples above on measles mention age, but factors such as nutritional status, immune competence, sex, ethnicity, access to treatment, concurrent chronic diseases, etc., etc., also play major roles.

Summary

The natural history of an infectious disease is usually studied in cohorts of patients who are followed over time. There is a potential risk for bias if only hospitalized patients are selected, since asymptomatic or mild cases will go undetected.

The study of incubation periods for diseases that are spread person to person requires careful chartering of the chain of transmission in the population.

Prognostic factors for the outcome of an infection are usually studied in cohorts as well, where clinical and laboratory findings early in the course of disease are compared with different outcomes.

The previous chapter showed that attack rate is associated with dose. There is also indication that higher dose may lead to more severe disease.

A large number of cofactors will influence the course of an infection once it has become established in a patient.

References

1. Panum PL. Observations made during the epidemic of measles on the Faroe Islands in the year 1846. Reprinted in Buck C, Llopis A, Nájera E, Terris M, editors:*The Challenge of Epidemiology.* Washington DC: Pan American Health Organization, Scientific Publication No. 505, 1989: 37–41.

2. Salas R, de Manzione N, Tesh RB, *et al.* Venezuelan haemorrhagic fever. *Lancet* 1991; **338**: 1033–36.

3. Hecht SR, Berger M. Right-sided endocarditis in infectious drug users. Prognostic factors in 102 episodes. *Ann Intern Med* 1992; **117**: 560–66.

4. Garenne M, Aaby P. Pattern of exposure and measles mortality in Senegal. *J Infect Dis* 1990; **161**: 1088–94.

15 Seroepidemiology

Which deals with serological tools for epidemiology, starting with an ultra-short description of the immune response and of laboratory methods. Titres and cut-offs are discussed, and there are some examples of seroepidemiological studies. Some potential biases are mentioned, in particular the age cohort effect.

For most diseases markers exist that can be measured in the laboratory, for example, for diabetes, thyrotoxicosis, myocardial infarction, renal failure, etc. Laboratory markers are of course also important in the diagnosis of many infectious diseases, such as the pattern of liver enzymes in hepatitis or the infected red blood cells in malaria. However, the use of serological markers of infection adds another dimension to laboratory diagnosis: they may not only tell us about the disease that the patient has at present, but also about diseases that he has had, in many instances decades ago, and from which he is now fully recovered. This gives an important tool for epidemiological studies.

When the body encounters a bacteria or a virus for the first time, a very complex immunological reaction is triggered to combat and control the spread of the pathogen. The details of this mechanism are being revealed in laboratories around the world at an amazing pace, and I will not go into any detailed discussion here; it could easily fill books considerably more voluminous than this one. I will just give a brief outline. Any substance that the immune system of the body recognizes as being foreign is called an *antigen*, i.e. something that generates an anti-reaction. It could be a protein, a polysaccharide, a lipid, or combinations of these. Usually, one does not call an entire bacteria an antigen, but rather each of its subcomponents. The immune system reacts to an antigen in two principal ways. One is called 'cellular immunity' and consists of the production of specific white blood cells capable of recognizing and destroying the particular antigen. The other works by the production of another type of white blood cells, called B lymphocytes, which produce specific proteins, called *antibodies* that bind to the antigen. This reaction is denoted the 'humoral immune response'. The binding may incapacitate the antigen, but also makes it easier for other white blood cells to destroy it.

The first type of immune response has relatively little clinical and epidemiological use. Cellular immunity has hitherto been difficult to assay, even if developments in this field are now rapid. The main use has been to test for exposure to tuberculosis bacteria: infection with *Mycobacterium tuberculosis*, or with its relatives such as the BCG vaccine, gives a cellular response that can be assessed by the injection of a small amount of purified antigen from killed mycobacteria just under the surface of the skin. Someone who has been infected with the tuberculosis bacteria or with BCG (or with a number of other mycobacteria that exist in our environment) will react to the injection with a small inflammation at the site. The size of this inflammatory reaction is believed to be correlated to the degree of immunological reaction.

On the other hand, the humoral immune response has acquired widespread clinical and epidemiological use. Several different classes of antibodies exist, but the two most important for epidemiology are called IgM and IgG ('Ig' stands for 'immunoglobulin'). This class division has to do with the overall structure of the antibodies, but within each class there exist huge numbers of antibodies with different *specificity*, i.e. that preferentially bind to different specific antigens. During and after an infection, the proportion of all antibodies that have a specificity for just the antigens of that pathogen will increase.

The presence and amount of antibody to an antigen can be measured in the laboratory: a test tube is coated with a small amount of the purified antigen from some external source. A serum sample from the patient is put in the same test tube. If there are antibodies directed against the antigen in the sample, they will bind. The test tube is then carefully washed to get rid of everything that does not bind to the antigen coat. Mark that there must be an excess of antigen in the tube, or some of the antibodies we want to measure will not find anywhere to bind, and will be washed out.

In order to visualize the amount of antibody that has bound to the coat, we need some marker. This is usually supplied by first injecting rabbits with human immunoglobulin (mixture of many different antibodies), which their immune system will recognize as foreign, and against which they will make their own rabbit antibodies. These anti-human rabbit antibodies are then taken out of the rabbit, and chemically bound to an enzyme that is able to convert some colourless substance into a coloured one.

The now enzyme-linked rabbit antibodies are put in the original test tube, and they will bind to the human antibodies that were already stuck to the antigen. After a renewed careful washing, a solution of the colourless chemical substance is put in the tube. The amount of substance that is converted by the enzyme into a coloured substance can be measured in a spectrophotometer. The photometer reading will be a measure of the amount of enzyme in the tube, and thus of the amount of anti-human rabbit antibodies, and thus of the amount of the antibody that we originally wanted to measure. This is a simplified description of a procedure called ELISA (enzyme-linked immunosorbent assay), which may also be done in other ways, and which is presently the standard way of measuring amount of antibody against a specific antigen.

Titres

The ELISA method can be used to directly get a quantitative value for the amount of antibody. Older serological methods, of which several exist, such as haemagglutination, haemagglutination inhibition, complement fixation, etc., usually only give a 'yes' or 'no' answer to the question whether there is antibody in the sample or not. With these methods, quantification is achieved by diluting the serum sample. One starts with a small amount of the undiluted sample (dilution 1:1). If this is positive for antibody, one takes another little volume of the sample and dilutes, most often 1:2 or 1:10. If this new sample is again positive, one tests the next dilution step, and so on until the last diluted sample was negative in the serological test. The highest dilution which tested positive is called the *titre*, and is taken as a quantitative value of the amount of antibody in the original sample. In the example given in Table 15.1 the titre would be 1:32 (sometimes given as the inverse, 32):

Note that a titre value of 1/1,000 is called *higher* than a value of 1/10, even though 0.001 is really smaller than 0.1.

The calculation of average titre for a group of subjects has to be done in a special fashion: since a dilution series like the one above gives a kind of exponential scale, with each step being twice as big

Table 15.1   *Example of results of antibody testing in a dilution series. (One often checks one dilution step 'extra', to make sure that the first negative titre was not just a laboratory error.)*

Dilution	Test result
1:1	+
1:2	+
1:4	+
1:8	+
1:16	+
1:32	+
1:64	-
1:128	-

as the previous one, one cannot just straightforwardly average the values to get a group mean. Instead one calculates the *geometrical mean titre* or *GMT*. An ordinary mean is defined as the sum of all values divided by the number of subjects, but a geometrical mean is attained by *multiplying* all the values, and then taking the *n*th *root* of this number, where *n* is the number of subjects.

If the titres in a group of four subjects were 1/32, 1/64, 1/32 and 1/128, the geometrical mean titre would thus be:

$$\text{GMT} = \sqrt[4]{\frac{1}{32} \times \frac{1}{64} \times \frac{1}{32} \times \frac{1}{128}} = \frac{1}{54}$$

Another way of performing the same calculation is to take the logarithms of each titre, adding them, dividing by number of subjects, and then exponentiating the result.

Sensitivity and specificity

One of the most important issues in serology concerns interpretation of borderline results. We touched upon this question in Chapter 7, but I will develop it somewhat here.

If a serological test always identified the correct antibody (high sensitivity) and never any other substances in the serum (high specificity), then there would be no problem. However, that is not the way reality works. Suppose we tested for antibody in a number of people that we knew had had a certain infection. The concentrations in their blood would not be exactly similar for them all, some would have high titres and some low. The pattern is often as illustrated in Fig. 15.1.

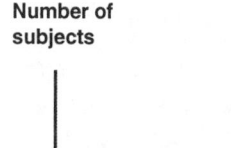

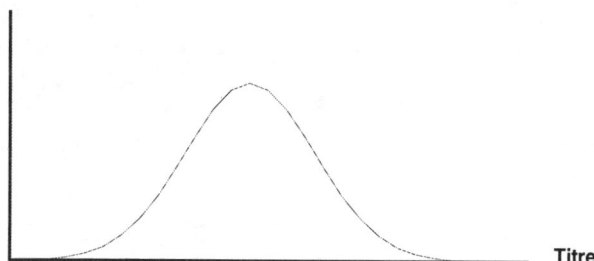

Fig. 15.1   *Example of distribution of antibody titres in a sample of immunized subjects.*

If we performed the same test on another sample of people whom we (in some mysterious way) knew had *not* had the disease, we would probably get the curve shown in Fig. 15.2.

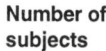

Fig. 15.2   *Example of distribution of non-specific titres in a sample of non-immunized subjects.*

The reason for this is that it is impossible to avoid unspecific reactions in a serological test. There will always be other proteins in serum that will stick to the antigen coat in the ELISA to some degree. This amount of unspecific reactivity will vary between individuals. If we now used this test in a real population, where some had antibody and some not, we would get a distribution of titre values that was a superimposition of the two curves (Fig. 15.3).

How should we deal with the titre values where the two distributions overlap? If we say that everyone with a titre value above **L** is seropositive, then we will include a number with strong unspecific reactions (high sensitivity, lower specificity). If we instead choose **H** as our *cut-off point*, then we will not get any unspecific reactions, but we will exclude some of the true seropositives (high specificity, lower sensitivity). In reality, also, the true shapes of the two curves are seldom known perfectly, and the size of the overlap zone will be uncertain.

Number of subjects

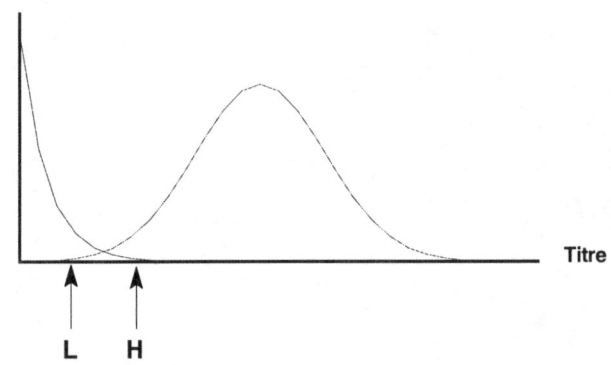

Fig. 15.3   Combined data for Figs. 15.1 and 15.2. L and H denote cut-off points.

There are no definite rules for choice of cut-off point, and it must depend on the reason for making the test. Reports from good serological studies should always include an account of how the cut-off point was set.

Time and titres

The different classes of immunoglobulins usually appear at different times during and after an infection. IgM antibodies can be detected first, but they also disappear from the patient's serum rather rapidly after the infection. IgG antibodies appear later, but usually remain in the serum much longer. This time pattern can sometimes be used to assess how recent an infection is, for example, IgM antibodies to hepatitis B virus are a certain diagnostic of acute infection.

Antibodies of the IgM type can seldom be detected earlier than one week to 10 days after the infection. IgG antibody titres may still be quite low during the acute disease. In these instances one makes used of so-called paired sera, where a new sample is taken some two weeks after the first one. If there is a clear increase in titre between these two tests, this is taken as indication or proof that the patient has had the infection in question. In most cases a four-fold raise in titre is required, for example from 1:16 in the first test to 1:64 in the second, but this rule may vary for different diseases. For some diseases, where titres in the general population are known to be low, a single high IgG-titre can be used to make a diagnosis: a titre against *Legionella* bacteria of more than 1:128 is often considered to indicate recent infection (at least if the patient has had symptoms suggestive of Legionnaire's disease).

Usage

There are two main uses of serology in epidemiology. The first is for descriptive, cross-sectional studies of seroprevalence in different populations. Such studies may then be rendered more analytical by relating seroprevalence to factors like age, geography, life-style, etc., and one example is given by the herpes simplex type 1 data described in Chapter 8, where an attempt was made to relate seroprevalence to changes in sexual behaviour. Another example comes from a Turkish study that tried to elucidate the risk factors for having become infected with hepatitis E virus.[1]

In a previous study of cardiovascular morbidity in five regions of Turkey, sera from 8,000 people had been collected together with demographic data from interviews. Out of these, 300 samples from each region were selected at random. Demographic data was missing for 51, and for some reason only 201 samples were used from one of the regions. The samples were tested with an ELISA in which the antigen had been produced by recombinant technique. Eighty of the 1,350 samples tested were positive for hepatitis E antibody, for an overall seroprevalence of 5.9%. Eight putative risk factors were then first analysed against seropositivity in a univariate analysis. Table 15.2 gives an example from this analysis, where the covariate studied was number of children.

Table 15.2   *Seropositivity by number of children in a study on hepatitis E markers in Turkey. Univariate analysis.*   Source: *Thomas* et al.[1]

No. of children	No. of subjects	% seropositive
0	497	3.4
1–2	481	5.2
>2	372	10.2

With the methods described in the previous chapters, we can calculate the ORs for being seropositive depending on number of children. The table is not set up in the usual 2×2 fashion, but it can easily be converted: in the first group, seroprevalence was 3.4%. If 497 is multiplied by 0.034, the result is 16.898, and we can thus guess that there were 17 seropositive and 480 seronegative in this group. Likewise, $481 \times 0.052 = 25.012$, so there were probably 25 positive and 456 negative in the group with one or two children. These figures are entered in a 2×2 table, the confidence interval is calculated according to the method for case-control studies in Chapter 4, and the *p* value can be calculated by the χ^2 method of Chapter 6. The group with more than two children is then compared with the baseline group in the same way. The resulting ORs, confidence intervals and *p* values are:

1–2 children versus none: OR = 1.5 (0.8, 3.1), $p = 0.171$
> 2 children versus none: OR = 3.2 (1.7, 6.2), $p < 0.001$

and there seems to be a strong association between 'having three children or more' and being seropositive.

The factors found to be significantly associated with seropositivity on the 5% level in the univariate analysis were: higher age, lower education level, higher number of children, having antibody to hepatitis C, and region of domicile. The authors then proceeded to make a logistic regression analysis, in which confounding will be controlled for, and found that number of children disappeared as significant risk factor. With all probability, this was due to confounding from age: younger persons generally have fewer children than older. The most interesting finding in this study was that no subject under age 20 was seropositive, whereas for hepatitis A, which is also an enteric infection, the large majority of people in Turkey will have antibody by age 20.

Another example comes from a study of hepatitis B infection among expatriates in South East Asia.[2] Prevalence of markers to hepatitis B infection was related to length of stay in South East Asia for 133 men. The result is shown in Table 15.3.

Risk for having become infected obviously increased with length of stay, and the incidence seems to have been around 10% per year of stay, but no attempt was made to control for confounders in this study, and we must assume that the men were similar in all respects apart from length of stay. The authors give heterosexual intercourse as the most probable source of infection. Only one in five of the infected gave a history of jaundice, so that if the study had been based on diagnosed cases only, the estimate of risk for infection would have been very different.

Table 15.3   *Prevalence of markers to hepatitis B virus (HBV) among expatriates in South East Asia.*   Source: *Dawson* et al.[2]

Length of stay (years)	Proportion with HBV markers	Percentage
< 1	0/11	0
1	2/22	9
2	6/34	18
3	3/19	16
4	9/19	47
≥5	12/28	43

The second usage of seroepidemiology is to follow incidence of an infection, either in a defined cohort or by repeated samples from a larger population. Incidence is then estimated from changes in prevalence between the samples. An advantage of seroepidemiology in this situation is that it obviates the need for continuous surveillance of cases: the cumulative incidence between two time points will be directly evident from the serological data. Also, subclinical cases will be included.

A somewhat different example of this method is given by the US study of a measles outbreak just after a blood drive already cited in Chapter 13.[3] During the months after a blood collection drive had taken place in a university in New England, a measles epidemic occurred in a couple of dormitories. Ninety students who had donated blood volunteered to take part in the study, among whom eight were clinically diagnosed cases of measles. You will remember from Chapter 13 that there was a strong association between pre-exposure antibody levels and risk of clinical disease. However, in this study the authors were also able to demonstrate a booster effect in already vaccinated students who did not develop clinical measles. Eighteen noncase students who had donated blood agreed to have their blood tested after the outbreak. The laboratory method used was 'plaque reduction test', which measures the degree to which the patient's serum is able to inhibit measles virus infection of a cell culture. Eleven of the 18 students who had antibody titres below 1,000 in their blood donation samples showed a four-fold or higher boost in titre after the outbreak, whereas none of the seven students with titres above 1,000 pre-exposure had a four-fold rise. This study is one of few to clearly demonstrate the existence of a booster effect, with rise in antibody titres after exposure in people who are already immune to a disease.

The issue of the importance of booster doses in maintaining immunity over long-term periods is controversial. It is receiving increased attention with the introduction of vaccine programmes that aim to eradicate diseases. Whereas previously immunized persons were still exposed to wild virus or bacteria circulating in society and thus had an opportunity to receive booster doses, in an eradication programme this re-exposure will disappear and the concern is whether the vaccine-induced immunity will still be lifelong.

Seroepidemiology is also used extensively in the evaluation of vaccine effects, as we shall see in Chapter 18.

Bias

Inevitably, many seroepidemiological studies are being performed on available material, i.e. most often frozen serum samples. There is always a risk of bias with this method. Who are the patients whose blood is saved in a serum bank? What was the reason for the test in the first place?

If one wants to make estimates of seropositivity in the general population, one should remember that sera in a serum bank were nearly always taken for clinical reasons. Patients who have a blood test taken differ from the general population in that they are ill somehow. The probability of visiting a physician varies greatly with age and sex, and in most developed countries a serum bank of random samples will be skewed towards older ages. Young women may have blood taken in connection with pregnancy, but men between 20 and 40 may not see a doctor for decades. Stored sera from children will often show a disproportionately high number of very young and of rather old children; the age groups when children can defend themselves but still not understand the necessity of the test will be underrepresented.

It is also dubious to what extent sera from healthy blood donors can be used to make population estimates. In countries where blood donation is unpaid, blood donors will probably tend to be healthier than the average person, whereas the reverse may be true in countries with paid donors. Few sociological studies have been made to characterize blood donors.

The age cohort effect

This is a rather special type of fallacy, which quite often pops up in seroepidemiological studies. If we test a random sample of the population for, say, antibody to *Helicobacter pylori*, and we find that seroprevalence increases with age, what does that tell us about present incidence in various age groups?

If a cohort of subjects were followed over time with repeated serologies, it would be easy to calculate the yearly incidence of infection. However, matters become more complicated if we instead choose to do a cross-sectional study right now, by measuring the percentage of seropositive persons in different age groups. For many diseases, like hepatitis A or herpes simplex type 1, such a study will show an increase of the proportion with markers (= seroprevalence) with increasing age. If those who are now 10 years old have a seroprevalence of 10% and those who are now 30 one of 35%, does this mean that 25% of today's 10-year olds will get the disease in the next twenty years? No, not necessarily. If the overall exposure to the pathogen is decreasing over time, perhaps as a consequence of improved hygiene, this means that those who have lived longer were more exposed when they were young. As an example, let us take an imaginary disease which is becoming rarer with time. Let us assume that up till 50 years ago the risk of catching this disease was 5% per year, if one was susceptible. After that, the risk has decreased by

% seroprevalence

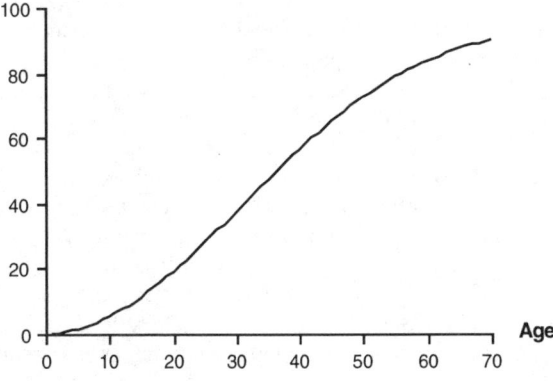

Fig. 15.4 *Example of seroprevalence versus age in a cross-sectional study.*

0.1% per year, so that it has been 0.1% during the last year. The present seroprevalence in the population would then be as Fig. 15.4 shows.

From this figure, it seems that the maximum age-specific incidence of this disease is for ages between 30 and 40, and that almost everyone will have had the disease when they reach age 70. In reality, the shape of the curve comes from the decreasing risk with time. What it shows is really that the older subjects were much more exposed when they were young. If the present incidence of 0.1% per year remained constant for the next 70 years the curve for a true cohort study of today's newborn would show an almost linear increase with age, and a cumulative incidence at age 70 of just under 7%.

This fallacy is known as the *age cohort effect* and is something to look out for whenever one uses a cross section of data from different age groups to make predictions about what will happen when the present-day population progresses through these age groups. For many Western countries, the age-curve for seroprevalence against hepatitis A looks something like the graph above, even though the incidence of hepatitis A is now quite low. Since there was more transmission of the infection several decades ago, the graph will display a sort of 'seroepidemiological archaeology'.

In the study from Turkey cited above, the authors point out that the peculiar age distribution of antibody to hepatitis E virus could be a cohort effect if transmission of this agent decreased sharply some 20 years ago.

Summary

Serology provides an important tool for infectious disease epidemiology, making it possible to measure incidence and cumulated incidence of infections in different populations.

Antibody levels are often given as titres, and these require special mathematics when groups are to be compared.

All serological tests suffer to a higher or lower degree from problems with unspecific reactions. By shifting the value for the cut-off point, one can increase either sensitivity or specificity (but not both).

Cross-sectional studies of seroprevalence can reveal risk factors for infection and suggest possible transmission routes, but cohort studies with frequent sampling of blood may be even more valuable in this respect, since time for seroconversion will be better described.

Collecting blood from a random population sample is always difficult, and it may be tempting to use stored serum samples instead. One should then be observant of the different biases possible.

The age-cohort effect is a special problem with cross-sectional studies in which seroprevalence is related to age. Has general exposure been decreasing with time? If so, the curve of prevalence for age will not show the age-dependent risk of infection facing the present-day population.

References

1. Thomas DL, Mahley RW, Badur S, Palaoglu KE, Quinn TC. Epidemiology of hepatitis E virus infection in Turkey. *Lancet* 1993; **341**: 1561–62.

2. Dawson DG, Spivey GH, Korelitz JJ, Schmidt RT. Hepatitis B: risk to expatriates in South East Asia. *Br Med J* 1987; **294**: 547.

3. Chen RT, Markowitz LE, Albrecht P, *et al.* Measles antibody: reevaluation of protective titers. *J Infect Dis* 1990; **162**: 1036–42.

16 The study of contact patterns

In which the concept of contact patterns is addressed in more depth. Methods to depict such patterns are described, and some examples are given of the research methods used to investigate how people mix

As has been pointed out repeatedly throughout this book, the epidemiology of infectious diseases is not only about the properties of various pathogens and their hosts but also to great extent an issue of contact patterns in the population. This is of course especially true for diseases that are spread from person to person, directly or via an intermediate host. In the prevaccination era, measles epidemics in Western Europe always started some weeks after school began in the autumn, and although it is difficult to prove, it seems highly likely that the increased contact density when children were again congregated after having been dispersed during the summer vacation was an important factor in this timing. It has been discussed why the incidence of most upper respiratory tract infections such as streptococcal angina, diphtheria and even meningococcal meningitis is always highest during the winter months. Some believe that the lower humidity of room air in winter makes the mucosal surfaces more vulnerable to attacks, but an equally plausible explanation is that people tend to meet at closer range indoors during the cold season, i.e. their contact pattern changes.

On the basic level, a person-to-person spread infectious disease cannot persist unless the infectious cases meet someone susceptible before they themselves have recovered. Taking the view of the pathogen, this means that an infection that is spread readily in daily social contacts does not have to be very long-lasting: an infectious case is almost certain to meet a susceptible within a day or two. However, for sexually transmitted infections contacts between a case and a new partner may be far between, and these infections thus have to have a very long period of infectivity, often in the order of months or years.

Continuing this line of reasoning, it seems improbable that the highly infectious and highly immunogenic (meaning leading to a very good protective immune response) diseases like measles or smallpox could have existed in human populations during the millenniums when we lived as hunters and gatherers. At that time, all humans lived in family or clan groups of maybe some 100 people at the most and with limited contact between groups.[1] If measles entered such a group, it would rapidly infect almost everyone, but where would the virus go after that? The probability of a contact outside the group during the infectious period must have been low. In fact, there exist modern data on measles epidemics in islands which indicate that a population of some 500,000 is necessary to maintain measles endemic.[2] The virus needs a steady influx of susceptibles, and in the absence of immigration this is supplied by the children who are born into the population.

For those diseases that can confer lifelong infectivity matters become different. The viruses of the herpes group, herpes simplex, varicella, etc., are sometimes reactivated in infected subjects, as cold sores or as shingles, which are both infectious, and those infections could thus persist in much smaller populations: someone infected with chicken pox as a child might develop shingles decades later, and subsequently infect his/her grandchildren in the group.

Incidentally, it is just those diseases that are highly infectious and immunogenic that we call childhood diseases. In a demographically stable society, the children are the only susceptibles entering the population, and they will be the ones who keep the chain of infection going. There is nothing about the viruses themselves that make them especially prone to infect young children.

Another interesting consequence of changing contact patterns in society is the shift towards higher average age at infection seen for many classical childhood diseases such as polio, hepatitis A, and possibly chicken pox. As hygiene improves and as families get less crowded, the amount of exposure during childhood decreases, and more and more children will escape infection. This will lead to an increased proportion of cases appearing in adolescents and adults, and these will often be more severe than if the infection had been acquired in childhood.

For many infectious diseases, population density, and subsequently contact density, thus become important determinants of epidemiology. However, even with a given contact density there may be considerable heterogeneity in contact patterns. As underlined in Chapter 10, it is a highly unrealistic assumption that everyone in the population has exactly the same chance of meeting everyone else. In order to better understand the epidemiology of infections, one also needs to study contact patterns.

Matrices and graphs

Sociologists often make use of graphs to describe the network of contacts in a group of people. They call them sociograms, and they could look like Fig. 16.1.

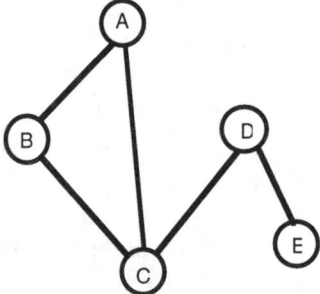

Fig. 16.1 *A sociogram, showing the contacts between five people.*

This graph could show which of the five people A, B, C, D and E knew each other. In the language of graph theory, the rings (people in this case) are called *nodes*, and the lines between them *links*.

An alternative way of representing the same graph would be to make a *contact matrix*:

	A	B	C	D	E
A	-	1	1	0	0
B	1	-	1	0	0
C	1	1	-	1	0
D	0	0	1	-	1
E	0	0	0	1	-

A 'one' shows that two people know each other, a 'zero' that they do not. The first row, or the first column, shows that A knows B and C, but not D and E.

This graph and this matrix are both *nondirected*, meaning that if A knows B, then B also knows A. If we had asked these five people who liked whom, the result may have been different(Fig. 16.2).

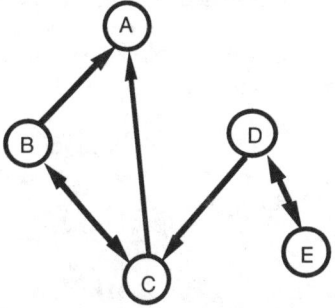

Fig.16.2 *An example of a directed sociogram, in which contacts may be unidirectional only.*

The graph shows that B and C both like A, as well as one another, etc., and the corresponding matrix would be:

| | | \| | To: | | | |
		A	B	C	D	E
	A	-	0	0	0	0
	B	1	-	1	0	0
From:	C	1	1	-	0	0
	D	0	0	1	-	1
	E	0	0	0	1	-

In this case, rows and columns are not equivalent, and this matrix should be read following a person's row from the left to see which of the others he/she likes. This graph and its corresponding matrix are both *directed*.

A problem with graphs like these is that they do not include times, and if the contact pattern is changing one would really need a series of graphs, maybe one for each day.

Contact patterns and infectious diseases

It is clear that graphs and matrices like these could be helpful for describing the spread of a disease in a population. There are, however, two rather distinct possible uses:
1. The first is the most obvious. It is when the exact path of an infection in a population is traced from person to person, and is

described in a directed graph, much as was shown in Fig. 10.2, introducing the concept of R_0. In analyses of outbreaks, such graphs are often useful, not least for presenting the results to other people afterwards. Several studies on the outcome of contact tracing for STDs include graphs showing the actual chain of infection. The nodes can be given different shapes or colour to denote the persons' sex, age, etc., and the links may be labelled with times or type of contact. Furthermore, the nodes need not be individuals, they could be subgroups of people, or as in some descriptions of influenza outbreaks, entire cities. We will call such descriptions of an actually occurring contact pattern *networks*.

2. The second usage is more subtle. It tries to describe the contact pattern in a population in the absence of any specific disease, the issue being to understand what would happen if a disease with a given attack rate was introduced: how far would it spread? Which would be its most likely path? Knowledge of contact patterns would also help clarify how endemic diseases remain in a population. Such a graph would most often not depict specific persons, but rather some type of average contact patterns, and often on different levels: contact patterns within families, between families, in schools, at work, etc. The links, also, need not be the actual contacts taking place, but rather the probability of contact within some time period.

For a population of any size, such a graph on the individual level would be impossible to construct. Instead, one would group people according to relevant characteristics and look at probability of contact between groups: what is the probability that a 24-year-old man has sexual contact with a 21-year-old woman? What is the rate of travel from city A to city B, and what would be the risk of an influenza epidemic in A spreading to B? Graphs of this kind form the basis of the stochastic models for infections described briefly in Chapter 10. We will call descriptions of this more general type of contact patterns *contact structures*.

In mathematical terms one could say that the contact structure is the set of all possible networks that could be observed, while a network is the one of all these possibilities that actually did occur. Methods to study contact patterns in real life, as well as the theoretical framework for analysing them, are still fields where much development remains, and this is one of the most important future research areas for infectious disease epidemiology.

Studying networks

The basic way of assessing networks is obviously to interview people about their contacts. The contacts named are then interviewed again, and so on, in order to get a bigger network. The size of the sample quickly becomes very large, but the approach may be possible for more restricted groups.

One such example concerning a disease that might be infectious comes from a study of the network between patients with the malignant lymphoma Hodgkin's disease in the area around Oxford in 1977.[3] It had been reported from the USA in the early 1970s that there seemed to be a high number of contacts between patients with Hodgkin's disease, which could support a role for some infectious agent with low attack rate and long incubation time. The relevant epidemiological question here is of course: what is a 'high number of contacts'? Compared to what? How does one know that there had been more contacts within this group of patients than within any random group in the population? The researchers in the Oxford study tried to answer this question in a type of case-control design. Ninety-seven patients diagnosed with Hodgkin's disease and reported to the regional cancer registry were identified as the cases. For each case, a control was chosen to be someone who had been admitted to a hospital in the region for any reason other than cancer or chronic disease at the same time as the case patient was diagnosed. The controls were also matched to the cases for sex, age, social class, and geographical area.

Eighty-seven of the cases, or a close relative if the case had died, could be interviewed about where they had gone to school and where they had worked. The obvious thing would then have been to ask all the controls the same questions. However, the investigators made a nice correction for possible recall bias in this study: if a case had died, they did not interview the corresponding control, but rather a close relative of the control, in order to make the collection of data as similar as possible.

A 'link' was then defined as an instance when any two people from this collection of 174 cases and controls had attended the same school or worked in the same workplace. If the findings from the American studies had been valid, there should have been more links between two Hodgkin's disease patients than between patients and controls or between two controls. In fact, it was calculated that the expected number of links between any 87 people in this group should be 40.75, and because there were found 40 observed links between the 87 Hodgkin's disease patients, this study showed little support for any infectious aetiology.

The method of asking people about their contacts becomes considerably more sensitive when sexual contacts are the issue, which is a somewhat paradoxical situation since this is probably the one area of infectious disease epidemiology where contact patterns are most important. An example of an attempt to elucidate a network of sexual contacts by the interview method comes from a study in Iceland.[4]

In 1987 there were 35 known HIV positive people in that country. Twenty-two of these agreed to participate in the study. They were asked to identify all their sexual contacts during the preceding seven years, including demographic characteristics (age, sex, residence, occupation, etc.), to describe the type of relationship they had had with them, and also to indicate if these partners knew each other and if so what kind of relationship existed between them. The reason for the last question was mainly to be able to collate the responses from all the subjects, making sure that the same person identified by two different subjects would not be counted as two.

The 22 subjects identified a total of 91 contacts. Sixty of these and 15 of the HIV positive subjects could be connected in a network, where every node was linked to at least one other. Seven of the HIV positive subjects could not be linked to any other infected person.

A small part of what the resulting network looked like is shown in Fig. 16.3. It is easy to understand that the description and analysis of networks such as these are far from straightforward.

The study of susceptible exposure attack rate in families requires careful elucidation of the actual networks of transmission, since it is important that the tertiary and higher order cases are differentiated from the true secondary ones. Another example is given by Panum's study in Chapter 14, where he needed to map out the exact network of the epidemic in order to calculate the incubation period.

Modern microbiology can sometimes supply tools to describe networks of infected people. This is done with some variant of 'genetic fingerprinting', by which individual strains of a bacteria or a virus can be traced through a group of patients. The most commonly used method is 'restriction-fragment length polymorphism' (RFLP), where the DNA of the pathogen is cut into pieces in a specific fashion by certain enzymes. The distribution of these split products can then be compared between samples from different patients by an electrophoresis method to see how similar they are.

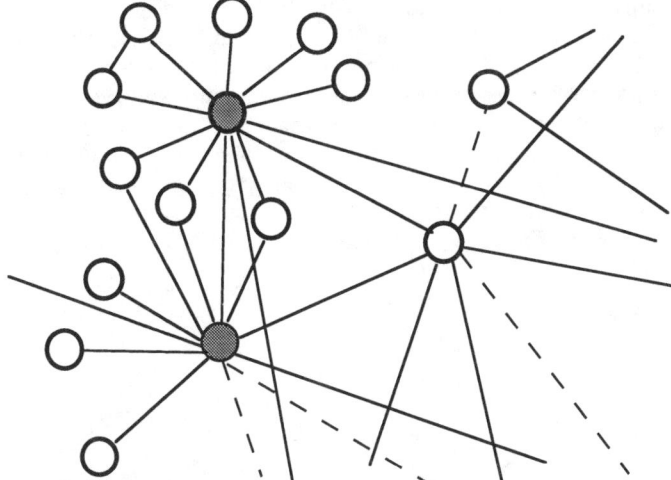

Fig. 16.3   *Part of a sociogram from a study on HIV positive people in Iceland. Shaded nodes denote HIV positive people, dashed links indicate uncertainty whether two people really had sexual contact.*   Source: *Haraldsdottgir et al.[4]*

Studying contact structures

Many important aspects of contact structures are obvious from everyday experience: people are more likely to meet someone living in their neighbourhood than someone living at the other end of the country. Schools and day-care centres make good mixing places for many infections. Social class and profession influence who meets whom to a great extent. Choice of sexual partner is often restricted to roughly the same age group as one's own.

The examples in the previous section showed how actual networks between individuals could be chartered. Data on contact structures could also be attained by interviews, and one example is given by surveys on sexual habits in random samples of a population.

In one such survey in Sweden,[5] a random sample of young adults were asked about their age at first sexual intercourse, and also about the age of their partner. The median age of the partners for each year of first intercourse was calculated for males and for females and the results are shown in Fig. 16.4.

In Fig. 16.4a, almost all the points fall on the line for equal age, showing that the men tended to have their first intercourse with someone who was their own age (in the median). Fig. 16.4b shows that the female subjects of the survey had had their first intercourse with a man who was about two years older than themselves. This simple survey thus revealed interesting differences in the two sexes' contact patterns at the beginning of sexual activity. One conclusion was that it must be unusual for young Swedes to have first intercourse with someone who has not had intercourse before, which should play a role for the epidemiology of sexually transmitted diseases in these young age groups.

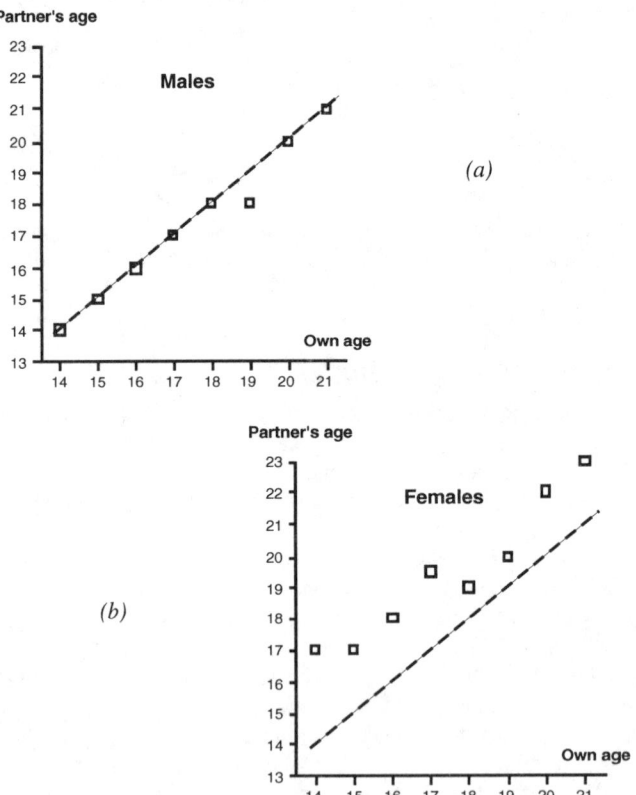

Fig. 16.4   *Results from a Swedish study, showing age at first intercourse versus that partner's age for male (a) and female (b) respondents. Broken lines indicate where the points should have been if both partners had been of equal age. From Giesecke et al,[5] with kind permission of the publisher.*

An interesting finding that emerges in virtually all surveys on sexual habits is that the average reported number of lifetime heterosexual partners is always higher for men than for women. Since a heterosexual intercourse involves one man and one woman, the total number of women partners reported by men should be the same as the total number of men partners reported by women. If there are equal numbers of the two sexes in the population, the average numbers should also be the same. This discrepancy has never been satisfactorily explained, even if sex-related propensity to over- or under-report number of partners could be one reason. Another explanation that has been suggested is that surveys tend to miss female sex-workers, who will have a very high number of partners, and who would raise the female average considerably if they had been included.

Rate of partner change

A central concept in epidemiological literature on sexually transmitted diseases is *rate of partner change*, or perhaps more appropriately *rate of partner acquisition*. This is defined as the average number of new partners that a person will have in a given time period, most often a year. It is thus just the same thing as **k**, the contact rate, in the formula for R_0 in Chapter 10.

There are, however, some problems with this concept as it is being used in research on STD spread. The principal one is whether this characteristic exists at all. Do all people have a rate of partner change, which could be given a value just like their age or height? The second problem is that even if we could assign a value for rate of partner change to a person, would this show any constancy over time? In the models discussed in Chapter 10, we just assumed an average contact rate for the population, or for large sub-populations, and this assumption could be valid even if individuals within that population changed their contact rate with time.

A person's rate of partner change is generally assessed in interviews, where people are asked how many partners they have had in the last year, last two years, last five years, etc. From such figures, one can get an estimate of the rate of acquisition of new partners. This is not straightforward, however, since one must take into account that partnerships could last across the boundaries of the time periods studied: if a person reports that he has had two partners in the last year, this could mean that he had two new partners, but equally well that one relationship ended and another commenced during the last year. If the previous relationship lasted 10 years, and the new one will also last 10 years, this person's rate of partner change would be 1/10 instead of 2. To get a slightly more reliable estimate, one usually subtracts the figure for partners in the last year from the figure for partners in last five years, and divides this by 4.

Regardless of the exact method of calculation, the problem with time constancy of the value remains. There is really no way of knowing that this figure will apply to the future behaviour of this person: a subject reporting a high rate of partner change could enter into a stable monogamous relationship tomorrow.

The next problem is that the actual figure is a poor descriptor of the actual contact pattern. A person X who reports two partners during the last year could have first had partner A and then partner B. If A was infected with an STD, this might be passed on to B via X. However, a not uncommon situation must be that the X had a continuing relationship with A during the year, and a short contact with B. He might even have ongoing sexual relationships with them both during the year. In the two latter cases, an STD could equally well be passed from B via X to A as the other way around. Matters could get even more problematic if the question in the interview was: 'How many new partners did you have last year?' A person who has had several ongoing relationships, but only with 'old' partners would answer 'zero' to this question. If his partners also had other partners, there would be a contact structure with high potential for spread of an STD in this group, even if almost all its members reported to have had no new partners during the year, and were thus assigned a rate of partner change of 0.

The epidemiologically more interesting question in the questionnaire would probably be: 'How many times during last year (last two, last five years) did you have sexual intercourse with someone who was not your partner in the previous intercourse?'

Type of mixing

Even if the concept of rate of partner change is quite problematic, it is still frequently used in STD epidemiology. This is due to the fact that different contact structures according to rate of partner change give rise to very different epidemic situations.

In the first instance, consider a situation where people having a given rate of partner change mostly or only have contacts with people with the same rate. Those who have a high rate would have contact with others with high rate, and those with low rate have contact with others with low rate. This pattern is called preferential or assortative mixing. If an STD entered this population, it would quickly spread among the high-rate people, but it may well be that the contact rate among large groups of the population was too low to sustain even an endemic level of the disease (using the terminology of Chapter 10, R_o would be below 1 in these groups). Cases of the disease in low-rate people would then mostly occur in those rare instances when a high-rate and a low-rate person had contact. The disease would only remain endemic within the group of people with high rates, and if this group was small compared to the total population, overall endemic prevalence could be low. A group of people who have a rate of partner change high enough to maintain an endemic of an STD is often called a *core group* in STD literature.

A second type of contact structure would be that rate of partner change did not influence choice of sexual partner at all. This is called random mixing. With such a contact structure, the initial spread of an STD would be much slower, since many of the infected would be low-rate subjects and would probably not pass on the disease. However, the final endemic prevalence of the disease could be higher than in preferential mixing scenario, since it could spread to much larger sections of the population.

Theoretically, there could also exist a type of contact structure with people actively seeking their partners from groups having a different rate of partner change from themselves: this is called dissortative mixing. From a sociological point of view, this seems like an improbable behaviour. Most of the human activities arranged to create contacts between people, such as bars, dance places, clubs, etc. try to bring kindred souls together. It is difficult to imagine a social arrangement aimed at bringing people together who were as dissimilar as possible.

The contact structure according to rate of partner change is very difficult to study in conventional surveys. Whilst data may be readily collected on the number of partners that the subjects themselves have had, we cannot usually reach these partners with the same question. However, the strategy of contact tracing for STDs offers a possibility to attain such data. In a study in Gothenburg in Sweden, 400 women with chlamydia infection were asked about their number of male partners in the last six months.[6] The distribution among these 400 women was:

1 partner	2 partners	3 partners	4 partners or more
228	135	32	5

From these 400 women, it was possible to contact 400 partners (for some of the women, no partner was found, for some more than one). These men were asked the same question, and their distribution on number of partners during the last 6 months was:

1 partner	2 partners	3 partners	4 partners or more
261	25	30	84

Let us just pause here for a moment to consider what these two samples represent. Is there any bias involved in choosing these 400 men and 400 women? The women were sampled out of a material of family planning and STD clinic attenders, and can be assumed to be representative of chlamydia-infected women in that population. The men, however, were sampled because they were reported as contacts. A man who has had contact with many women must have a higher probability of being named as a contact than one who has only had sex with one woman. The distribution of the 400 men in the study on reported number of partners above will thus be skewed to include 'too many' men who have had a high number of partners. This quite evident from the much higher figure for men than for women reporting four partners or more.

This means that a contact matrix for these 800 people can only be interpreted for the women, i.e. the matrix below should only be read along the lines from the left:

		\multicolumn{4}{c}{Men}			

		\multicolumn{4}{c}{No. of partners last 6 months}	
		1	**2**	**3**	**≥ 4**	
Women	**1**	180	5	9	34	228
No. of	**2**	69	16	14	36	135
partners	**3**	9	3	7	13	32
last 6 months	**≥ 4**	3	1	0	1	5
		261	25	30	84	400

Thus, there were e.g. 135 women who reported two partners in the last six months. Among partners of women in that group, 69 had only had that woman as a partner, 16 had had one more, 14 had had two more women, etc.

If women showed exclusive preferential mixing, all the figures of the above table should have been on the diagonal from upper left to lower right, since a woman would only choose a partner with her own rate of partner change. If on the other hand mixing had been completely at random, the distribution along each of the four lines should have been similar, and equal to the total distribution in the line at the bottom, since all women should choose among the men in the same fashion, regardless of their own rate of partner change.

This is a good point to recapitulate the ideas behind the χ^2 test introduced in Chapter 6: for each of the cells in the table above we could calculate an expected value, *if* the women's choice of sexual partner had been at random. For the top line, we see that a total of 228 women reported one partner. If choice had been at random, these 228 relationships should be divided on the four rows just like the bottom line. There should thus be:

$$228 \times \frac{261}{400} = 149 \text{ women in the top left hand corner,}$$

$$228 \times \frac{25}{400} = 14 \text{ in the second cell of the first line}$$

$$228 \times \frac{30}{400} = 17 \text{ in the third, and}$$

$$228 \times \frac{84}{400} = 48 \text{ in the top right hand cell}$$

If we perform this calculation of *expected* (assuming random choice of partner) number in each cell of the table, and then subtract these values from the corresponding value of the actual table, the result becomes:

Difference between observed and expected number in each cell:

		Men			
		1	**2**	**3**	**≥ 4**
	1	31	– 9	– 8	– 14
	2	– 19	8	4	8
Women	**3**	– 12	1	5	6
	≥ 4	0	1	0	0

With some imagination, one could see a tendency for the high positive values to concentrate on the diagonal, implying that women more often choose a man with about equal rate of partner change than would be expected just by random choice. That the distribution of the observed table is unlikely to be at random can be proven by calculating the actual χ^2 value, which gives a $p < 0.01$.

Random sampling of networks

Since the actual network of contacts in a population of any size is almost impossible to describe, one would need some method to get a representative sample of networks, from which a better understanding of the contact pattern could be attained. One such interesting strategy makes use of a kind of random walk in a network, and the method has been used to study the population of Canberra, Australia.[7]

One starts with a list of all the people in the population. From this list, a number of persons are chosen at random, and each of these subjects are interviewed, and asked to list all their contacts. From each person's list, one contact is chosen at random, and this person is also approached and interviewed about all his/her contacts. The process could go on for an arbitrary number of steps. If resources are available only for a certain number of interviews, one has to decide whether to choose a larger group of primary subjects and restrict the interviews to secondary contacts, or to choose a smaller group initially and continue to tertiary or higher-order contacts. The first choice gives better precision in describing the average person-centred network, whereas the second choice increases the power to detect more complicated networks in the population.

In the Canberra study it was decided to select 60 people out of a total of around 200,000 as primary subjects, and to go on to tertiary contacts. A total of 180 people were thus interviewed. They reported on average 30 links with other people in Canberra, and by asking about age, sex, occupation, etc., it became possible to describe the person-centred networks in more detailed fashion: of all reported links, 8% were to relatives, 25% to current or former neighbours, and 24% to work associates. It is interesting that as many as 67% of all links were directed, i.e. A reported B as a contact, but B did not mention A.

Obviously, there will be a number of people who are listed by more than one subject of the study. These were generally not interviewed, but by combining the lists of all the interviewees it was possible to link some 6,000 people in Canberra in a large network where everyone was connected to at least one other person and where the maximum distance between any two people was six links. The core of this network obviously included the persons interviewed (since only they had listed all their contacts), but also of 274 other persons named by two or more study subjects, and one could speculate that the characteristics of these should be of great interest for the understanding of infection spread in a population such as this.

Summary

Contact patterns play an important role for the shape of epidemics and endemics. On the most basic level, frequency of contact decides which diseases could persist in a population.

Even with a given average contact rate, there may be large variations between subgroups. Simple epidemic models usually assume random mixing in the population, but this is unrealistic for most diseases.

Contact patterns can be described with methods borrowed form sociology: graphs and contact matrices. A network describes the actual pattern of contacts between a group of individuals, whilst a contact structure tries to describe the probability of contact between groups of individuals with certain characteristics.

The basic research method for investigating contact patterns is the interview or survey. However, subtyping of bacteria or viruses may sometimes make it possible to reconstruct the exact network through which an infection has spread.

The rate of partner change is an important concept in theoretical STD epidemiology, but its validity is unclear. Different types of mixing with regard to rate of partner change will have implications for the rate of spread and final endemic level of an infection.

References

1. McKeown T. *The Origins of Human Disease.* Oxford: Blackwell Publications, 1988.

2. Black FL. Measles endemicity in insular populations: critical community size and its evolutionary implication. *J Theor Biol* 1966; **11**: 207–11.

3. Smith PG, Kinlen LJ, Pike MC, Jones A, Harris R. Contacts between young patients with Hodgkin's disease. *Lancet* 1977; **2**: 59–62.

4. Haraldsdottgir S, Gupta S, Anderson RM. Preliminary studies of sexual networks in a male homosexual community in Iceland. *J AIDS* 1992; **5**: 374–81.

5. Giesecke J, Scalia-Tomba G-P, Göthberg M, Tüll P. Sexual behaviour related to the spread of STDs – a population-based survey. *Int J STD AIDS* 1992; **3**: 255–60.

6. Ramstedt K, Giesecke J, Forssman L, Granath F. Choice of sexual partner according to rate of partner change and social class of the partners. *Int J STD AIDS* 1991; **2**: 428–31.

7. Klovdahl AS. Sampling social networks: a simple approach to a difficult problem. Abstract from *Workshop on Generalizability Questions for Snowball Sampling and other Ascending Methodologies.* University of Groningen, Feb. 20–21, 1992.

17 Methods to decide whether or not an illness is infectious

One of the most challenging tasks of infectious diseases epidemiology is to try to decide if a disease is infectious or not. This chapter looks into some methods devised to investigate this problem. The most common method is to look for clusters in space and/or time, but an example of an ecological study is also given. Also, one example is given of the converse: searching for a disease for a newly found microbe.

The series of experimental steps required to prove that a pathogen is the cause of a specific disease were first laid down by a German microbiologist called Löffler in 1883.[1] Thoughts along the same lines had been published by Henle in the 1840s and by Klebs in 1877. Löffler's boss was another well-known microbiologist called Koch, who had also advanced similar thoughts, and the rules have become known to posterity as *Koch's postulates*: they are often cited in slightly different versions, but Löffler's original wording was:

The fulfilment of these postulates is necessary in order to demonstrate strictly the parasitic nature of a disease:
1. The organism must be shown to be constantly present in characteristic form and arrangement in the diseased tissue.
2. The organism which, from its behaviour appears to be responsible for the disease, must be isolated and grown in pure culture.
3. The pure culture must be shown to induce the disease experimentally.

Even though the postulates are still being cited today, they are too dependent on bacteriological methods to be really useful. Nevertheless, it would probably be fair to say that most infectious disease clinicians and microbiologists still feel uneasy with calling a disease infectious on purely epidemiological grounds, they want to see and characterize the responsible microbe first.

The general idea behind epidemiological studies that aim to find out if a disease is infectious is the following: if a disease can be transmitted from one person to another, then cases should tend to cluster in space and in time. We have already seen an example of such a study in the previous chapter, where links between cases of Hodgkin's disease were compared to links among controls. If that disease was infectious it should be possible to observe clusters of patients, but no such clustering was found in that study.

A good example of a cluster analysis comes from a study of the skin disease pityriasis rosea in the UK.[2] During a two-year period in the late 1970s all general practitioners within the catchment area of the skin department at North Staffordshire Hospital Centre were asked to refer all suspect cases of pityriasis rosea. One hundred and twenty-six patients had the diagnosis confirmed, and they were asked about date of onset of rash and place of residence.

A list of all possible pairs or two patients was subsequently made. The first patient was paired to each of the other 125, the second to each of the remaining 124, and so on. For all such pairs of patients the distance between their houses and the time period between the respective onsets of disease was calculated. The number of all possible pairs between n subjects is $n(n-1)/2$, so in this case distances in geography and in time had to be calculated for $126 \times 125 / 2 = 7,875$ pairs of patients. The reasoning then goes as follows: if the disease was *not* infectious, then there should be no correlation at all between distance in time and distance in geography. The cases would appear at random in the population, and a plot of time distance versus geographical distance for each pair would look just like a shotgun swarm.

However, if the disease did have an infectious aetiology, then there would be a structure in such a plot, in that cases who lived close together would also have dates of onset quite near one another. There might be several different chains of infection going on simultaneously in the area, but these would be spread at random, and within each chain, cases would tend to cluster in space and time. Alternatively, only one chain of infection could have been operating during the two-year period, but then cases would appear further and further from the original source as time progressed. In both instances, a plot of time distance versus geographical distance for all pairs would tend to show a pattern with the points falling around a line from lower left corner to upper right corner of the diagram.

In this study, a simple 2×2 analysis was performed by grouping the pairs into those who lived more or less than 250 metres part, and into those who had dates of onset more or less than 14 days apart:

	$\leq$ 250 m	> 250 m	
$\leq$ **14 days**	10	338	348
> **14 days**	69	7458	7527
	79	7796	7875

The expected number of cases in the upper, left-hand cell would be $79 \times 348 / 7875 = 3.5$, which is clearly lower than the 10 observed. The p value was less than 0.005, and this result thus supports that pityriasis rosea might be transmissible.

Another example of cluster analysis, which this time fails to find any clusters, comes from a UK government report looking into the disease bovine spongiform encephalopathy.[3] When 'mad cow disease' as it was also called was first diagnosed in the late 1980s, there was considerable worry about the possibility of spread to humans. The disease was assumed to have entered the cattle population of the UK by feeding the animals leftovers from slaughtered sheep. A very similar disease in sheep, scrapie, has been described since at least the 18th century, and the agent responsible for scrapie could have been transmitted to cattle in this way.

There are also a number of spongiform encephalopathies that occur in humans, and at least two of them, kuru and Creutzfeldt-Jacob's disease (CJD), have been shown to be transmissible. Kuru was discovered in New Guinea, and the route of transmission was shown to be the ceremonial handling and ingestion of human brains afflicted by the disease. Transmission of CJD has been shown to occur via neurosurgical instruments, via corneal transplants, and via injection of human growth hormone extracted from cadaver pituitary glands.

The reasoning in the report goes as follows: if scrapie could be transmitted to humans and appear as CJD or a similar condition, then CJD should be more common in populations living near herds of sheep with high prevalence of scrapie. In fact the incidence of CJD is strikingly uniform all over the world; it is a very rare disease with an incidence of 0.5–1 per million population per year. It shows the same incidence in the UK, where scrapie had been endemic for at least 250 years, as in Japan where scrapie is rare, and in Australia, where scrapie is nonexistent. The authors also cite a French study, which fails to find any association between local scrapie prevalence and CJD incidence in different regions of France.

This kind of meta-analysis or review of a number of published studies provides an interesting philosophical problem, and one which occurs not infrequently in everyday life. The data seem to indicate a lack of transmission of scrapie to humans, but what degree of certainty can we attach to this finding? What is the p value? How low could the risk be and still not be detected in studies such as these? Part of the problem is a lack of a specific hypothesis, such as 'What is the highest risk of transmission of scrapie to humans commensurate with the observed data?'. However, life is full of incomplete answers to imprecise questions, and at some point, science fails us and we must rely on common sense. Just as in clinical medicine, where a lot of the things we do probably have frail scientific foundations, the control and prevention of infectious diseases in everyday life cannot always stem out of impeccable scientific studies, or wait for one to be undertaken. There is nothing wrong with relying on common sense as long as one is aware of what one is doing, and also ready to rethink in the light of new data.

There exists a long list of diseases for which an infectious aetiology has been postulated. One of the most intensely researched is multiple sclerosis, which seems to have some connection with measles, although it is still uncertain how. Several studies implicate infection with coxsackie virus as at least one triggering factor in the development of diabetes. Two diseases that are receiving a lot of attention when this book is being written are sarcoidosis and Crohn's disease. However, for most such diseases with a suspected infectious aetiology the research will be arduous: long incubation times, low transmission risks, and perhaps genetic influences on disease expression are all factors that make the epidemiology of an infection difficult to elucidate.

As a general point about cluster analysis, it should be pointed out that even if cases of a disease tend to cluster in space and/or time, this does not prove that it is infectious. Many other kinds of exposures could be brief and localized, and would thus also tend to create clusters of cases. In fact, this is probably true for most environmental exposures.

Ecological studies

All the studies cited so far in this book have focused on individuals. This may seem like a strange statement, since, as was stated in the first chapter, epidemiology is about assigning people to different groups. By observing group-defining characteristics of patients, we are trying to see further than the individual patient, hoping that knowledge of their age, sex, geographical area, behaviour, etc., will aid in diagnosis, treatment and prognosis, and also in the elucidation of risk factors and aetiologies.

However, in all previous examples, the exposures and the outcomes were measured for individuals. Knowledge of the individual's exposures (where this term is again used in a very general sense, and also includes such factors as gender and age), helps us to assign people to the different groups we want to compare and study. Epidemiology is about comparing groups, but the composition of the groups comes from measurements on individuals.

A different approach is used when entire populations are compared, with little or no knowledge about the individual risk factors and outcomes in those populations. A good example of such an *ecological study* comes from the observation that colon cancer is much more common in Western Europe, where people eat very little fibre, than it is in Central African countries, where people eat lots of fibre. In such a study, the average fibre intake in two populations is compared, and also the incidence of colon cancer in these two populations. Only the two populations as a whole are studied: we know nothing about the individual fibre intake or the individual risk of colon cancer in the two areas. It could be that those who developed colon cancer in Europe happened to eat as much fibre as the average African even if mean European intake was low.

An example of an ecological study that tried to elucidate a possible infectious aetiology for a form of cancer comes from a multicentre project involving 17 populations from 13 different countries.[4]

The bacteria *Helicobacter pylori* was discovered in Australia in the early 1980s. It soon became clear that infection of the stomach wall with this bacteria played a role for the development of gastritis and ulcers. Some studies also indicated an association between infection with *Helicobacter pylori* and cancer of the stomach. In order to further clarify this association, the investigators collected blood samples from some 200 members from each of 17 different populations. These persons were chosen a random from population-based registers, from general practitioner's lists, from drivers' licence rosters, or from health-screening programmes. The aim was to get 50 samples each from men and women aged 25–34 and 55–64 years, and subjects who declined to participate were replaced by someone else in the same age and sex-group.

The sera were assayed for antibody to *Helicobacter pylori*, and these results were compared to published national statistics on mortality rates for gastric cancer. Findings of ecological studies are often presented as so-called scatter plots (Fig. 17.1).

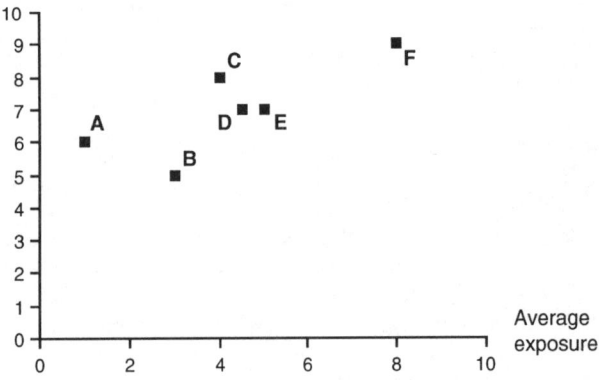

Fig. 17.1   Invented example of how the results from an ecological study are usually presented. Each labelled point represents one population, for which an average exposure and an average outcome measure can be assessed.

A regression line is then fitted to the data, and tested for statistical significance as described in Chapter 8. In this study, the values on the *x* axis were the proportion of the randomly tested subjects in each population with antibody to *Helicobacter pylori* and the values on the *y* axis were the published death rate from gastric cancer in the corresponding country. The authors found a strongly significant association between these two values, and they state that in a population where everyone was infected with *Helicobacter pylori*, there would be a six-fold higher risk of gastric cancer compared to a population where seroprevalence was zero.

One only has to think about ecological studies for a moment to realize that their major problem is confounding. They compare populations that may differ in many ways apart from the one factor under study.

There must be a number of factors that are different between populations of Central Africa and Western Europe, apart from their intake of fibre.

A somewhat different ecological study, which made clever use of registry data, indicated that some sexually transmitted agent may play a role in the development of cancer of the cervix.[5]

Two data sets were used: the yearly notified cases of gonorrhoea in the UK from the mid-1920s to the mid-1970s, and the yearly reported mortality from cervical cancer in women born between 1902 and 1947. Ordinarily, data on cancer incidence or mortality is presented per calendar year, but in this study the author wanted to compare total mortality between age cohorts followed over longer periods. All women in the UK were thus grouped into cohorts with the women who were born 1900–1904 in one cohort, those born 1905–1909 in the next, etc. Mortality from cervical cancer was then only compared between all the cohorts when the women in each cohort were of the same age, i.e. mortality from cervical cancer in women aged 35–39 was compared for all the cohorts, and then mortality in women aged 40–44, and so on. Obviously, to be able to perform this calculation one needs data on year of birth for all the women who died of cervical cancer. The mortality within each cohort was then averaged for all the five-year intervals along that cohort's life to give a kind of mortality rate for that cohort.

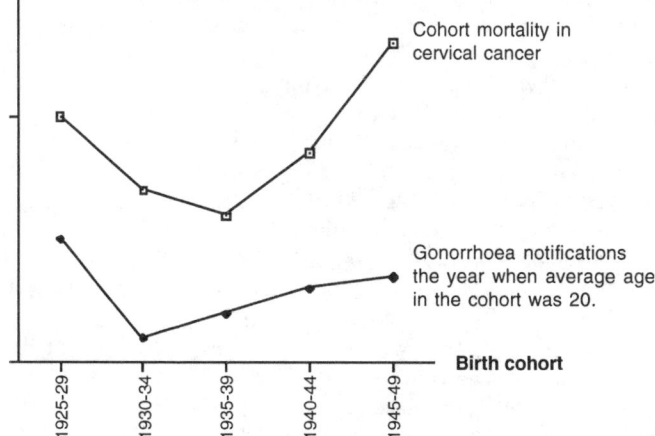

Fig. 17.2   *Mortality in cervical cancer and national reported gonorrhoea incidence the year when average age in cohort was 20 for five successive cohorts of women in the UK. (Disregard scales on y axis.)*   Source: *Beral[5]*

Age-specific incidence data for gonorrhoea did not exist for most of the period, but the author observed that for the years when age was registered incidence always seemed highest in women aged around 20. The assumption was thus made that each woman was at peak risk of acquiring gonorrhoea at age 20, and that this risk was equal to reported overall gonorrhoea incidence in the year when she turned 20.

For each cohort of women, two curves were plotted in the same diagram: the first was mortality rate for that cohort and the second was reported gonorrhoea incidence at the time when average age within that cohort was 20. The principle is shown in Fig. 17.2.

The author demonstrated a correlation between risk of gonorrhoea in young adulthood and subsequent risk of cervical cancer, and since it seemed unlikely that the gonorrhoea infection would be carcinogenic in itself, it should rather be regarded as a marker for some other, unknown sexually transmitted agent which showed the same incidence pattern. Several epidemiological studies now implicate infection with human papilloma virus to be strongly associated with cervical cancer.

Newly discovered pathogens

The connection between a pathogen and a disease often starts with the discovery of a new pathogen in a number of patients with a common disease pattern. This was the way most of the bacteria were coupled to their diseases in the golden era of microbiology at the end of the last century, when the people mentioned in the first paragraph of this chapter worked. A more recent example is given by the bacteria *Helicobacter pylori* mentioned above, and one of its discoverers actually tried to fulfil Koch's postulate by drinking a suspension of the bacteria and observing the symptoms. (He did develop subjective as well as a biopsy-proven gastritis.)

Another example comes from the finding of a new organism called CLB (coccidian-like or cyanobacterium-like body) in patients with diarrhoea.[6] The organism was first detected by microscopy in HIV patients, in people with a history of foreign travel, and in a small outbreak at a hospital in Chicago. However, human faeces contains a vast number of microbes, and just because a new one is discovered in diarrhoea patients this does not mean that it is causally associated with the disease. One first step to establish an aetiological role for CLB would be to find an endemic area for the organism and demonstrate that it is more common in people with diarrhoea than in healthy subjects.

This study was carried out among foreign residents and tourists in Nepal. Since 1989, stool samples from such patients with diarrhoea attending either of two outpatient clinics in Kathmandu had been routinely examined for CLB. Incidence had seemed highest during the summer months, and it was decided to carry out a prospective case-control study in the summer of 1992.

In order to group subjects into cases and controls one needs a case definition. The one used here defined diarrhoea as:
• a change in the normal pattern of bowel movements, and
• at least three loose stools during 24 hours.

This is a quite common case definition for diarrhoea, but you will find others in the literature.

Controls were chosen among other attendants of the clinics. They should meet the following criteria:
• no history of diarrhoeal illness during the preceding two weeks
• no history of a CLB infection
• being able to provide a stool sample.

In previous examples in this book we have just defined the cases, assuming that all who did not meet this definition could be controls. Here, the authors also made a control definition, which is a good idea when the exact spectrum of disease is unknown and one wants to sharpen the distinction between cases and controls as much as possible. CLB was detected in the stools of 108 out of 964 patients with diarrhoea (11%), but only in one of 96 control patients (1%). The p value for this difference can be calculated by the $\chi2$ method, since the *expected* values for all four cells will be higher than 5, and was found to be p = 0.003.

Next, the authors proceeded to look for risk factors for being infected with CLB, and they then made another case-control study, where the cases were now 93 patients diagnosed with CLB infection compared to the 95 CLB-free controls. The groups had similar age and sex distributions, and the proportions of tourists versus long-term residents were the same. All those 188 people were asked about travel in Nepal during the week prior to the clinic visit, about drinking untreated water, swimming, eating fruits and vegetables, about water systems in their residence, etc. Of these variables, only drinking untreated water was significantly associated with infection: 17 of the 93 cases versus five of 94 controls (one control obviously did not answer this question). Water samples were also analysed from the homes of 22 cases, and in one of these CLB was found.

When the resident subjects were asked about how long they had lived in Nepal, it was found that median length of stay for the cases was 11 months (inter-quartile range 4–21), but for the controls 24 months (range 9–72). The difference was highly significant and could point to some kind of immunity to the infection developing with time. In comparisons such as these, it is wise to use the median instead of the mean, since just one person with a very long stay would influence the mean disproportionately.

This study thus shows a strong association between the finding of CLB in faeces and diarrhoea. If one wants to be puristic, there may still be uncertainty about its aetiological role: the organism could still just be a marker of risk if it happened to exist in the environment in the same milieu as the real cause. However, this pathogen should also still be undiscovered, since the CLB cases had the same pattern of other enteric pathogens (*Shigella*, *Salmonella*, *Giardia*, etc.) as the healthy controls, and an overall prevalence of any such pathogen less than half of the non-CLB diarrhoea cases.

Summary

Several epidemiological methods exist to investigate whether or not a disease has an infectious aetiology. The basic idea is to look for clusters in time and space, which could indicate transmission from infectious to susceptible. If cases show more links than could be expected, or if cases that appear close in space also appear close in time, there is some evidence for transmission. However, it should be remembered that several environmental exposures also will be localized, so that cases may appear clustered.

For many diseases with a suspected infectious aetiology the demonstration of this fact could be made more difficult by long incubation periods, low transmission risk, and strong influence of other cofactors.

Ecological studies can provide a starting point for clarifying an infectious aetiology, but all such studies have problems with confounding.

The connection of a newly found pathogen to a specific disease pattern is best achieved by fruitful collaboration between the microbiologist and the epidemiologist. Case-control studies provide a useful tool for elucidating risk factors, which can then be looked into more systematically.

References

1. Löffler F. *Mitteilungen aus den Kaiserliche Gesundheitsamt.* Vol II, 1884. Translation taken from Brock DT. *Robert Koch. A Life in Medicine and Bacteriology.* Madison, Wisconsin: Science Tech Publishers, 1988: 180.

2. Messenger AG, Knox EG, Summerly R, Muston HL, Ilderton E. Case clustering in pityriasis rosea: support for role of an infective agent. *Br Med J* 1982: **284**: 371–73.

3. Ministry of Agriculture, Fisheries and Food. *Report of the Working Party on Bovine Spongiform Encephalopathy.* London: HMSO, 1989.

4. The Eurogast Study Group. An international association between *Helicobacter pylori* infection and gastric cancer. *Lancet* 1993; **341**: 1359–62.

5. Beral V. Cancer of the cervix: a sexually transmitted infection? *Lancet* 1974; **1**: 1037–40.

6. Hoge CW, Shlim DR, Rajah R, *et al.* Epidemiology of diarrhoeal illness associated with coccidian-like organism among travellers and foreign residents in Nepal. *Lancet* 1993; **341**: 1175–79.

18 The epidemiology of vaccination

Here the study of the protection afforded by vaccination is discussed. The concept of vaccine efficacy is introduced, and the difference between direct and indirect effects explained. The implications on study design of various interpretations of a figure for vaccine efficacy gets a mention.

The concept of immunity and the measurement of vaccine-induced immunity are central to infectious disease epidemiology, and really have few counterparts in the study of noninfectious diseases. The fact that some people are resistant to exposures that would always cause disease in others rarely applies to factors such as diets, toxins, or radiation. It is true that there may be genetic differences in susceptibility to other harmful exposures, but these are generally poorly understood, and in most instances there is little evidence of the all-or-nothing effect of immunity on susceptibility to infections.

The other aspect of vaccine-induced protection that is particular to infectious disease epidemiology is that vaccination, at least in most instances, not only protects the vaccinated subject, but also the people around him, in that their exposure to the pathogen will diminish. If enough people are vaccinated in the population, the amount of exposure to the still unvaccinated will decrease to a point where epidemics can no longer be sustained, and we will have herd immunity in that population just as discussed in Chapter 10. This concept of *indirect protection* from other people being vaccinated is important when one wants to measure the effect of a vaccine on individuals, as we shall see below.

Vaccine efficacy

The ideal way to measure the protective effect, or efficacy, of a vaccine is to perform a regular randomized, controlled clinical trial, where one group of subjects is given the real vaccine and another is given placebo. The two halves of the cohort are then followed over time, and the number of cases counted. The incidence rates are calculated for both groups, dividing the number of cases by the number of person-months or person-years in each group.

If the incidence in vaccinated is called I_v and in unvaccinated I_u, then the *vaccine efficacy* is defined as

$$VE = \frac{I_u - I_v}{I_u} \times 100 \quad (\%)$$

That is, if the vaccine gives total protection there will be no cases at all in the vaccinated group, which means that I_v will be zero, and VE $= I_u/I_u \times 100 = 100\%$. If the vaccine is useless, incidence will be the same in both groups and VE $= 0$.

When vaccine efficacy is assessed in an outbreak situation, the respective attack rates are usually substituted for the incidence rates in the definition of VE.

Different types of studies

A cohort study

One example of a study to measure vaccine efficacy comes from a trial of a *Haemophilus influenzae* type b (HIb) vaccine in the USA.[1]

The entire cohort consisted of 61,080 children who came for a well-care visit to any of 16 centres within a medical care programme in northern California between 1988 and 1990. In order to be included, the children had to have at least one visit before six months of age, and infants with known immunodeficiencies were excluded. A complete vaccination consisted of three doses of vaccine during the first year of life. In this study, the subjects were not randomized to receive treatment and no placebo was used. Children born during the first week of each month were not offered vaccination, and they constituted part of the control group. The other part of the control group was made up of children to parents who were offered vaccination but declined.

In order to study the efficacy of a full vaccination, follow-up of vaccinated children to diagnose HIb infections only started one week after the third dose. Since the third dose was given at age eight months on average, an age bias would have been introduced if all infections in the control group had been recorded. Follow-up of a control child thus started when the child was one week older than the average age at which the vaccinated children received their third dose. The children in both groups were followed till age 18 months. Cases of invasive HIb infection (meningitis, cellulitis, bacteraemia) were detected by several different routes: weekly reports from nurses at the study centres, monthly listings from the microbiological laboratory of positive HIb cultures from normally sterile sites, discharge notes from hospitals in the area compatible with HIb disease, and requests for reimbursement of hospitalisations outside the area.

In total 20,800 infants received a full vaccination, and they were compared to 18,862 unvaccinated children who were also followed from age 255 days up till 18 months. The number of person-years in the two groups were 12,949 and 11,335, respectively. There were 12 cases of severe HIb disease in the unvaccinated children, versus none in the vaccinated group. In this case, I_u would thus be 12/11,335 and I_v would be 0/12,949. Vaccine efficacy would be estimated to be 100%. The confidence interval for this estimate must be calculated by a Poisson method which we have not covered in this book, but the authors give the lower 95% bound for the VE to be 68%.

Since this was not a randomized trial, extra care must be taken in excluding possible biases. If, for some reason, the vaccinated children had been at lower risk of HIb infection than the children in the control group, then the estimated VE would be too high. The report presents a number of indications that this was not the case, the most valid being that incidence in the control group was no higher than among all children at the participating centres during the years preceding the study, and also lower than the concurrent incidence among the children in the area not taking part in the study.

The authors justify the chosen design with two arguments, one being that it is logistically difficult and time-consuming to undertake a randomized study of this size, the other that there was an increasing demand for HIb vaccination among the parents in the area during the period. This last argument points to a possible confounder: with all probability, the better educated parents will be the ones who will demand vaccination first, and if risk of severe disease is associated with social class, there may have been a lower incidence among the children in the treatment group even in the absence of vaccination.

A case-control study

An important theoretical paper from 1984[2] pointed out the possibility of using a case-control design in attempts to measure vaccine efficacy. This approach was used in a study of meningococcal vaccine in Brazil.[3]

One hundred and thirty-seven cases of bacteriologically confirmed meningitis with *Neisseria meningitidis* serogroup B occurring in children aged three to 83 months were collected in São Paulo during 1990 and 1991. For each child, four controls were selected, matched on age and neighbourhood. The controls were recruited in a very hands-on fashion with the interviewer starting in front of the residence of the case and walking to the first house to the left, inquiring about children of appropriate age in the household. The interviewer then continued to call on houses down the street to the end of the block, and if this was not enough to recruit four controls, he returned to the starting point and proceeded to the right along the street. As a last resort, the interviewer went around the entire block in an anticlockwise direction.

In a case-control design, the objective is to assess whether there is any difference between the proportions vaccinated in the case group and the control group. If all cases are unvaccinated and all controls vaccinated, this would obviously indicate that the vaccine has a protective effect. In this study, vaccination status of cases and controls was determined solely from vaccination cards given to the mothers at vaccination; all children with indefinite vaccination status were excluded from the analysis.

Of the original 137 cases, it was not possible to select controls for 10, and for another 15 vaccination status was indefinite. Four hundred and nine controls had definite vaccination status, and they were matched to the 112 remaining cases. Sixty-eight of the cases (61%) had been vaccinated, versus 260 of the controls (64%).

If you look back at the definition of VE above, you can see that

$$VE = \frac{I_u - I_v}{I_u} = 1 - \frac{I_v}{I_u} = 1 - RR$$

where RR is the relative risk for disease in vaccinated compared to unvaccinated. An obvious extension of this formula to the case-control situation is to substitute OR for RR. In this study, the OR for being vaccinated according to disease status can be calculated from the 2×2 table:

	Vaccinated	Not vaccinated	
Meningitis	68	44	112
Control	260	149	409
	328	193	521

The value becomes $(68 \times 149)/(260 \times 44) = 0.89$, and the estimated vaccine efficacy would thus be $(1 - 0.89) \times 100 = 11\%$. This is not very impressive, but the authors then went on to show that age at vaccination seemed very important, and that the VE in children aged more than four years when they are vaccinated was as high as 73%.

A crucial prerequisite for all non-randomized studies of vaccine efficacy is that there is no difference in exposure between the two groups: vaccination must be completely at random regarding future risk for disease. A good example of a situation where an estimate like the ones above would be totally misleading comes from the present Swedish strategy for BCG vaccination. General BCG vaccination was abandoned in 1975, and after that the aim has been to only offer the vaccine to children at increased risk of tuberculosis. These are mainly children to immigrants from countries where TB is still much more common than in Sweden. If this selection of higher-risk children could be perfected to be totally accurate (100% sensitivity in identifying children who might later be infected with TB) and the vaccine has less than 100% efficacy, then *all* the cases of TB in Sweden in the future will appear in vaccinated children. Someone who was ignorant about this bias in vaccination might regard such a finding as an indication of very poor VE.

A somewhat different randomized, controlled trial

An alternative study design was used in another trial of meningococcal vaccine, this time in Norway.[4] Instead of randomly allocating vaccine or placebo to individual subjects, the unit of randomization was school. Since meningococcal disease in Norway shows one peak for the age group 13–21, it was decided to undertake the study in 1,335 secondary schools, where the pupils were 14–16 years old. Each school was randomized to receive either vaccine or placebo to give to all its participating students, and the investigators, school nurses and students were all blind as to the content of each school's batch. Seventy-four percent of all Norwegian pupils in the age group agreed to participate. The vaccine group consisted of 88,000 pupils in 690 schools, and the placebo group of 83,000 students in 645 schools.

A full vaccination comprised two injections, and cases of meningococcal disease among the participants were counted only if they occurred more than two weeks after the second injection. Cases were chiefly ascertained through the well-performing laboratory reporting system previously set up in Norway.

During the study period, there were 89 confirmed cases of group B meningococcal disease in the age group. Sixty-three of these had been pupils of secondary schools. Thirty-nine of these were participants of the study, but one of these had the disease before study start and two fell ill less than two weeks after the second injection (both these pupils were later found to have received placebo). Since the unit of randomization was school, individual cases should not be counted, but rather school outbreaks. However, all cases except two were singular.

There were 11 outbreaks (12 cases) in the 690 vaccine schools versus 24 outbreaks in the 645 placebo schools. The 'per school incidence' was thus $11/690 = 0.016$ versus $24/645 = 0.037$, and the vaccine efficacy measured on school-basis would be

$$VE = 1 - 0.016/0.037 = 57\%$$

The difference between the two groups of schools can be shown to have a *p* value of 0.012 with Fisher's exact test (which was here performed one-sided, since there was no reason to believe that the vaccine efficacy would be negative).

The authors conclude that this VE is too low to justify a general vaccination against meningococcal group B infections in Norway, since the yearly incidence is just around 200 cases. A very different conclusion from quite similar numerical findings could be made from a study of an oral typhoid vaccine in Indonesia:[5] the estimated VE for this vaccine was also only around 50%, but the incidence of typhoid in the country is so high that 250,000 cases per year could theoretically be prevented by a vaccination programme with good coverage.

Direct versus indirect protection

The Norwegian study above is interesting also from another aspect than the block randomization, and that has to do with indirect protection: during outbreaks of meningococcal infections there will be a high prevalence of healthy carriers in the population; many times higher than the proportion who actually fall ill. In an outbreak in a military camp in Sweden some years ago, meningococci could be isolated from the throats of over half the soldiers. Even during nonepidemic periods, some 5% of young adults in Northern countries are healthy carriers.

As was discussed briefly at the beginning of this chapter, vaccines offer protection not only to the vaccinated, but also to the people that they might otherwise have infected. At least, this is true if the vaccine protects against infection as well as disease, and in fact, many bacterial vaccines seem to also protect against carriage. If this was the case with the vaccine used in the Norwegian study, exposure would have been lower in the vaccine schools than in the placebo schools, since there would have been fewer carriers in the former group. The classic definition of vaccine efficacy assumes that the degree of exposure is similar in the vaccinated and unvaccinated groups, and does not take into account such indirect effects. However, it may well be argued that the figure measured in this study is more interesting from a public health point of view, giving an estimate of the population effect of a vaccination programme. The combined direct and indirect protection of a programme is sometimes referred to as its *effectiveness*.

The implications of different study designs could be shown by the following schematic diagrams. First assume that all subjects within one population (a school, a town, or a country) are vaccinated, whilst another, similar population serves as the control group (Fig. 18.1).

It is quite evident that exposure would be lower in the population on the left, and a vaccine efficacy according to the formula above would be an overestimate.

If we instead vaccinate half the subjects of a given population, the situation would be as shown in Fig. 18.2.

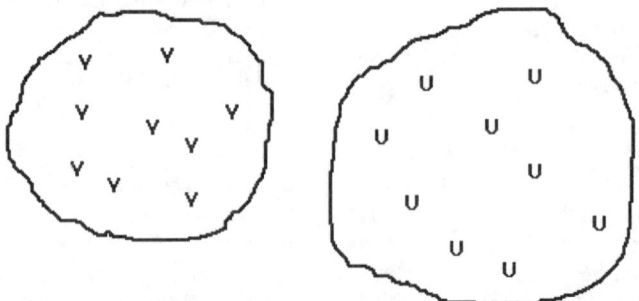

Fig. 18.1 *A vaccine trial comparing one totally vaccinated (V) and one totally unvaccinated (U) population.*

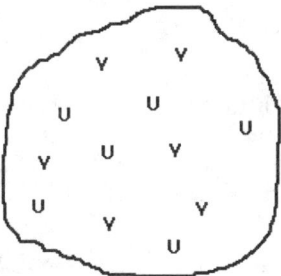

Fig. 18.2 *A vaccine trial in which vaccinated (V) and unvaccinated (U) subjects can mix freely.*

In this case, at least if vaccinated and unvaccinated mixed freely, exposure would be the same to both groups, and the VE would be valid. You should note, however, that in this situation exposure of unvaccinated will also decrease, so that overall incidence will be lower than before the vaccine was introduced. If the study was designed to detect a certain difference in incidence between the groups, one may well find that one gets fewer cases in the control group than was anticipated based on pre-trial data, and the study findings may not achieve the statistical significance one had hoped for.

Assessing effectiveness by surveillance

The ultimate way of assessing the overall effectiveness of a large-scale vaccination programme is obviously by observing a clear decrease in incidence of disease. One nice example of rapid effect comes from the introduction of HIb vaccine in Finland.[6]

The trials of one type of vaccine started in 1986-87 when three doses were offered to 50% of all infants, group allocation being by date of birth. In 1988–89, two two-dose vaccines were compared, each being given to 50% of all infants, and since 1990 another type of two-dose vaccine has been offered to all infants. The authors maintain that all cases of HIb meningitis treated in hospital in Helsinki since at least the early 1970s have been recorded, and that fairly reliable data are available back to the late 1940s. Actual age for each of these cases was not known, but from good surveillance data from the period 1984–90, they can postulate that 90% of the cases should have been in the 0–4 years old group.

Since the population of the Helsinki area was increasing during this period, the yearly number of cases has to be divided by the actual number of newborn to four year-olds to get comparable incidence figures. The results for four five-year periods with good data are given in Table 18.1.

This study may have been performed a bit early, since the vaccination programme had hardly begun to have any effect in the last five-year period, but there does seem to be a break in a previously upward trend. Another important piece of information in the article is that there was not one single case of HIb meningitis in the age group in the Helsinki area in 1991.

Table 18.1 *Incidence of* Haemophilus influenzae *type b meningitis in Helsinki from 1946 to 1990. Incidence in children under five is estimated.* Source: *Peltola* et al.[6]

5-year period	Cases total	annual	Population of 0–4 year-olds	Yearly incidence per 100,000 0–4 year olds*
1946–1950	36	7	39,900	16
1966–1970	65	13	51,800	23
1976–1980	117	23	49,500	43
1986–1990	68	14	51,800	24

* Assuming that 90% of all cases were in this age group

Evaluation by serology

As you can see from the US and Norwegian examples above, modern cohort studies of vaccine efficacy tend to become quite big. This is due to the fact that even if severe HIb and meningococcal infections are important public health problems, incidence is still quite low. In the US study, 0.6 unvaccinated children per 1,000 had severe infections during the study period, and in the Norwegian study only 0.3 per 1,000. Especially if the vaccine efficacy is a bit lower than 100%, such incidence figures will necessitate large groups to attain any significant differences. One alternative, quicker approach is to resort to serological methods, and measure the levels of antibody to the vaccine postvaccination. Ideally, the antibody measured should be protective, not just a marker of seroconversion, and there should also be some defined titre that is known to be protective. The VE would then be estimated as the proportion of a vaccinated group that acquire protective levels of antibody after vaccination.

Such serological methods are often used also to follow the waning effect of a vaccination: in the absence of any natural or man-made boosters, the level of any antibody will decay with time. When the titre falls below the protective level the vaccination is assumed to no longer be protective, and estimates of the average time from vaccination till loss of protective antibody levels have been used in various vaccination programmes to determine when a booster dose is needed.

In a study of hepatitis B vaccination in The Gambia, 1,041 children were recruited into a cohort[7] with the intention of giving everyone at least three injections during the first year of life. The clearly protective level of hepatitis B virus surface antibody (anti-HBs) is usually assumed to be more than 100 international units (IU) per litre, whilst a level of less than 10 IU/litre is considered to indicate lack of protection. Subjects with anti-HBs values between 10 and 100 IU/litre probably have some protection.

The problem with any study of a vaccine that requires more than one dose is to get all the study subjects fully vaccinated. There will always be those who just had one dose, or two, and the question is how these should be accounted for. In a regular clinical trial of a vaccine, they would most often be excluded, but when one tries to assess a vaccination programme rather than just the vaccine itself, they should be included. This will give a better estimate of how the vaccine will perform in the more routine health care situation. In the Gambia study, only 87% of the children had received three or four doses of the vaccine during their first year of life, but results were analysed for all children who had had at least one dose. At age one, 763 children who had not had a natural hepatitis B infection could be traced and tested for antibody, and of those 92% had a level over 100 IU/litre, 6 % between 100 and 10, and 2% below 10. Serology would thus indicate that the VE was at least 92%, and maybe as high as 98%.

The mean antibody level decreased by 75% from age one to two, and by another 28% from age two to three. Such rapid decline in antibody during the year after the vaccination is seen for most vaccines, but need only cause concern if nonprotective levels are reached too soon, and in fact the proportion of unprotected children increased only slightly: at age two only 4% had anti-HBs below 10 IU/litre, and at age three, 5%.

Nineteen out of 698 vaccinated children tested at age three showed serological markers of having had a natural hepatitis B infection, although none of them had demonstrated any clinical signs of hepatitis. Five of these still had an acute or chronic infection with positive HBsAg, but of these two were probably infected by their mothers at birth, one had a proven and one a probable postvaccination level less than 10, and one had a level of 57 IU/litre in the first year. The remaining 14 had just seroconverted in anti-HBc antibody, which showed that they probably had had a natural infection, and several of these had had postvaccination titres of protection well over 100 IU/litre. These results thus show that one should be careful in assuming that generally accepted protective levels of after vaccination always do protect against infection. As for most other laboratory values in medicine, biological variation is important and the significance of an individual figure may be different for different persons.

Another study, which indirectly questioned the validity of commonly assumed cut-off values for protective titres, was performed in Sweden to assess the need for booster diphtheria vaccination in children.[8] Diphtheria antitoxin levels were measured in six-, 10-, and 16-year old children who had been given three doses in infancy. The issue of the study was to see by how much titres had declined and by how much they could be boosted by an additional shot, but it also provided data on prebooster protective levels. It was found that the children who had the three doses at ages three, four and a half, and 15 months had significantly higher remaining titres than those who had them at ages three, four and a half, and six months. Of the children who received the more condensed schedule, as many as 48% had titres below the protective level before receiving a booster at age 10. Another study also showed very low titres in adults. However, at about the same time in 1984, there was the first outbreak of diphtheria in Sweden since the late 1950s, with 17 diagnosed cases. Most of the patients were elderly men with alcohol problems, and only one case occurred in a child. There was very little evidence of spread to a more general population, even though a high proportion seemed to lack protection and the validity of the cut-off values assumed for protection would thus seem dubious.

What does a figure for VE mean?

The concept of vaccine efficacy as explained above seems quite straightforward, being a measure of how much incidence (or attack rate) decreases in vaccinated subjects. There are, however, two quite different ways of interpreting a figure of, say, 80% efficacy for a certain vaccine:

1. Either it means that 80% of the vaccinated get total protection against the infection, and the remaining 20% get none, or

2. All vaccinated decrease their susceptibility to infection by 80%.

Another way of expressing the second alternative is to say that everyone vaccinated is protected against 80% of all possible exposures.

In any clinical trial of vaccine efficacy, the difference between these two interpretations becomes very important, and for many commonly used vaccines it is not known which type of protection they confer. The problem comes from the time that the vaccinated and unvaccinated groups are followed in the study. If the vaccine is one that gives total protection for a proportion of the vaccinated but none for the rest, it will not matter how long the study runs. The estimated figure for efficacy will tend to be correct in short trials as well as in long ones, even if the precision of the estimate will of course be better in a longer trial. However, if the vaccine works by increasing the minimum dose of the pathogen needed for infection, this means that just by chance the probability of anyone vaccinated encountering a high enough dose to cause infection will increase with time. For such vaccines, the calculated VE will depend on the time the subjects are followed, and it will decrease with the length of the study. Furthermore, estimates of VE will be different in different countries: in a country with high general levels of exposure the efficacy will seem lower than in a country with low levels.

This difference in mode of action will also be very relevant when one wants to evaluate how soon booster vaccinations need to be given after a primary immunization: is a perceived increase in incidence in vaccinated with time due to waning immunity, or is it just a sign of a vaccine effect of type 2 above?

Herd immunity and eradication

Discussions about vaccine coverage often make use of the concepts introduced in Chapter 10 on modelling. The most important of these was already discussed there, namely the relation between basic reproduction rate and the vaccine coverage necessary for herd immunity. You will remember that the minimum proportion, p, of the population that needs to be immunized in order to attain herd immunity is given by the formula:

$$p > 1 - \frac{1}{R_o}$$

so that the higher the basic reproductive rate, the closer one will have to be to total immunization coverage.

Notice that I used the word 'immunized' and not 'vaccinated' in the sentence above. The latter word is usually taken to mean those who were injected with the vaccine, whereas the former refers to those in whom the vaccine actually worked. A vaccination coverage of 100% will thus only have an *immunization* coverage equal to the VE of the specific vaccine.

The issue of herd immunity through vaccination is of course intimately linked to the possibility of *eradication* of an infectious disease. If the actual reproductive rate in the population can be kept below 1 long enough, the disease will eventually vanish. (Obviously this last statement is only true for infections that are spread exclusively between humans. It seems unlikely that diseases like plague, salmonella, tick-borne encephalitis or influenza will ever be eradicated.)

Considerations about R_o and about maximum vaccine coverage achievable in a programme are thus very important and real aspects of public health strategy.

Another nontrivial effect of large-scale vaccination programmes is that average age at infection will be shifted upwards. This also follows from the concepts introduced in Chapter 10: when a high proportion of the population are immune, the risk for a susceptible to meet an infectious will decrease. If every 100th contact is infectious instead of every 10th, average time until one meets an infectious case will obviously increase. This means that diseases which were previously almost exclusively childhood infections will start appearing in adolescents and adults. In some instances, only the *proportion* of cases that appear in adults will increase, whereas the total number of adult infections will decrease, since overall incidence is falling. In other situations there may, however, be a true increase in adult incidence.

One very important example is given by vaccinations against rubella: the reason to vaccinate children against rubella is not to protect them against infection which is anyway quite mild in most cases, but rather to protect women from an infection during pregnancy, which may lead to congenital malformations in their child. In the absence of vaccination, the majority of women will have acquired immunity before they reach fertile age, and the objective of a vaccination programme would be to further decrease the proportion of susceptible pregnant women. However, some vaccination schedules might even increase this proportion. Just consider what happens when the vaccine is first introduced: usually a programme will start with immunizing all infants born a certain year, and then successive birth cohorts during the following years. The slightly older siblings will not be vaccinated, but will be subjected to diminished exposure from their immunized younger brothers and sisters. There will thus be an age cohort consisting of the children who were some one to five years old when the programme started who will reach adolescence with considerably lower prevalence of immunity than their older or younger siblings.

This very dangerous effect of the programme will eventually disappear, some 40 years after the start of the programme (when all women who become pregnant will have been vaccinated), but a continuing uptake below herd immunity level might still increase the number of susceptible pregnant women. Some countries started their rubella vaccine programmes by just immunizing girls at the age of 12, but considerations like these have led to a change in policy to vaccinate all children. A further consequence of this reasoning is that rubella vaccination programmes should not be started in a country where an uptake corresponding at least to herd immunity level cannot be guaranteed.

Summary

The study of vaccinations is an important branch of infectious disease epidemiology. Vaccine efficacy is defined as the percentage reduction of incidence in vaccinated compared to unvaccinated. It does not, however, take into account the reduction in exposure caused by diminishing incidence in vaccinated people around the study subjects, i.e. the indirect effects of vaccination.

For vaccine studies in which subjects are not randomized to vaccine or placebo it is crucial that there is no difference in exposure between the two groups. If this can be shown to hold, case-control studies may provide a quicker and easier way to measure vaccine efficacy.

Since vaccine studies assessing actual incidence tend to be big and lengthy projects, an often used alternative is to measure antibody levels in vaccinated subjects. The problem here is to be certain of exactly which kind of antibodies, and which levels, correspond to protection.

For many vaccines it is unclear whether the figure for efficacy denotes the proportion of the vaccinated that will get total protection, or an overall reduction in susceptibility provided to all vaccinated. This difference has important implications for the design of studies to measure vaccine efficacy, especially as regards the length of the study.

With vaccine-maintained herd immunity, it may be possible to eradicate certain infectious diseases. However, large-scale vaccination programmes will shift the age distribution of cases, which especially in the case of rubella might have serious consequences.

References

1. Black SB, Shinefield HR, Fireman B, *et al*. Efficacy in infancy of oligosaccharide conjugate *Haemophilus influenzae* type b (HbOC) vaccine in a United States population of 61 080 children. *Pediatr Infect Dis J* 1991; **10**: 97–104.

2. Smith PG, Rodrigues LC, Fine PEM. Assessment of the protective efficacy of vaccines against common diseases using case-control and cohort studies. *Int J Epidemiol* 1984; **13**: 87–93.

3. De Moraes JC, Perkins BA, Camargo MCC, *et al*. Protective efficacy of a serogroup B meningococcal vaccine in São Paulo, Brazil. *Lancet* 1992; **340**: 1074–78.

4. Bjune G, Høiby EA, Grønnesby JK, *et al*. Effect of outer membrane vesicle vaccine against group B meningococcal disease in Norway. *Lancet* 1991; **338**: 1093–96.

5. Simanjuntak CH, Paleologo FP, Punjabi NH, *et al*. Oral immunisation against typhoid fever in Indonesia with Ty21a vaccine. *Lancet* 1991; **338**: 1055–59.

6. Peltola H, Kilpi T, Anttila M. Rapid disappearance of *Haemophilus influenzae* type b meningitis after routine childhood immunisation with conjugate vaccines. *Lancet* 1992; **340**: 592–94.

7. Chotard J, Inskip HM, Hall AJ, *et al*. The Gambia hepatitis intervention study: Follow-up of a cohort of children vaccinated against hepatitis B. *J Infect Dis* 1992; **166**: 764–68.

8. Mark A, Christenson B, Granström M, *et al*. Immunity and immunization of children against diphtheria in Sweden. *Eur J Clin Microbiol Infect Dis* 1989; **8**: 214–19.

19   The epidemiology of HIV infection and AIDS

Here many of the methodological problems touched upon in the previous chapters are again discussed by examples from the study of the epidemiology of AIDS and HIV infection.

The epidemiology of AIDS is rather more complex than the epidemiology of most other infectious diseases. It highlights most of the methodological problems discussed in the previous chapters, and this is the reason that I have put this chapter at the end of the book as a recapitulation.

Short background

The new disease 'acquired immunodeficiency syndrome' was first described in 1981, and a system for notification was set up shortly thereafter, first in the USA by the Centers for Disease Control (CDC), and subsequently in other countries. As underlined in the discussion of outbreaks in Chapter 11, such a surveillance requires a case definition, and the CDC published a list of symptoms and diseases that should define a case of AIDS. This list contained a number of so-called opportunistic infections, i.e. infections with pathogens that do not cause disease in otherwise healthy people, and a number of malignancies. The two most important case-defining conditions were pneumonia caused by the protozoon *Pneumocystis carinii* and the vascular skin tumour Kaposi's sarcoma.

The first years' surveillance indicated that the disease mainly afflicted men who had had sexual intercourse with other men, people who had been in contact with Haiti and with Africa, and people who had received a blood transfusion. During these years, there was much debate about the aetiology of AIDS, and many theories were advanced. One was that semen itself was immunodepressive, especially in anal intercourse, another that repeated exposure to many pathogens, mainly the virus CMV, led to an exhaustion of the immune system. The study on the association between poppers and AIDS has already been mentioned in Chapter 4.

Even though epidemiological research revealed strong risk factors, such as unprotected anal intercourse with many partners, one could not say that epidemiological science managed to establish that AIDS was an infectious disease. However, in 1984 the human immunodeficiency virus was isolated, and its role in the pathogenesis of AIDS became clear. Tests for antibody to HIV were available for use in the clinic from 1985, and they showed that many people were infected with the virus without having any symptoms of AIDS. At about the same time it became possible to test for the virus itself in infected people, and the Western blot was introduced. This test analyses the exact pattern of antibody response in seropositive people and makes it possible to decide if this is a true infection or just an unspecific reaction in the tested person. The polymerase chain reaction (PCR), which discovers minute amounts of viral genome, was first used to test for HIV infection in the late 1980s.

In the early years of the epidemic it was believed that only a small percentage of those infected with HIV would go on to develop AIDS, but with time the estimate of this proportion has increased, and it now seems that most infected individuals will eventually develop the disease.

Incidence/prevalence

One of the major problems for AIDS epidemiology has been to get an idea of the number of people infected with HIV in a country, and also to measure the rate of spread of the virus. Already in the mid-1980s it was clear from clinical follow-ups, as well as from HIV tests of stored blood samples, that the time from infection with HIV to the development of AIDS must be several years on average. A notification scheme for AIDS will thus not show the actual incidence of HIV infection in a country, but rather the incidence of several years ago.

This is another example of the problem with subclinical infections discussed in Chapter 11 on surveillance. Most people who are infected with HIV will not notice it, and they will not come to a clinic to be diagnosed and notified. About one third of those infected actually do experience an acute viral illness a few weeks after the infection, with fever, sore throat, and sometimes a rash, but this is generally too mild or too unspecific to lead to a diagnosis.

The only certain way to assess the prevalence of HIV infection in a country would thus be to test a representative sample of the population for HIV antibody. However, even since the epidemic was first recognized, many people have had a very adequate personal anxiety of being found seropositive, and members of already stigmatized groups such as homosexual men and injecting drug users have feared registration by the authorities. The number of people who would choose to abstain from such a test would probably be too large to make the result valid. This is especially true for most industrialized countries, where overall prevalence has been low, and where the result of testing even a large sample would be difficult to interpret if just a few persons declined.

As an alternative strategy it has been suggested to test people who come into contact with the health-care system, and who are either asked directly to provide a sample for HIV testing, or whose blood is drawn for other tests, but could also be used to look for HIV antibody. (Since most countries now agree that it is unethical to test people for HIV infection without their knowledge, the latter option requires that all identifying information linking a test result to a person is first removed from the blood specimen.) Examples of such groups are blood donors, hospital patients in general, and pregnant women. However, there are problems with selection bias for each of these groups:

1. Potential blood donors are explicitly asked about a number of factors and behaviours that correlate to the risk of being HIV positive, and if they admit to these factors or behaviours, they are not allowed to donate blood. This means that there will be an under-representation of people at risk among blood donors. Also, we know little about what characterizes blood donors compared to the general population.

2. The age distribution of patients in hospital is heavily skewed towards higher ages. Even if blood samples from outpatients were included, the group of men between adolescence and 40 would still be very much under-represented. Young women at least come in contact with the health-care system for reasons of contraception or pregnancy, but men of similar age may not see a physician for decades. Obviously, sera from patients will also include a disproportionate share of people who are ill for other reasons,

and it is not clear how this relates to HIV prevalence.

3. Pregnant women are probably the most representative of these three groups, since some 80–90% of all women have at least one child during their lifetimes. Again, though, it is uncertain how the probability of being pregnant relates to the risk of being HIV-positive. Take past infections with sexually transmitted diseases as an example: such episodes increase the risk that a woman will be infertile, but there is also a positive association between past STDs and the probability of being HIV positive. This means that HIV prevalence may well be higher in those women who do not become pregnant.

All these are examples of selection bias, as we discussed in Chapter 5. None of the three groups is quite representative of the general population, and the HIV prevalence in any of these groups cannot be assumed to be equal to overall prevalence.

Measuring *incidence* of HIV infection is even more difficult. The only certain way would be to have good yearly estimates of prevalence, and to calculate changes between them. This is being done in subpopulations of countries, for example, in some regions in Africa, or in the US Armed Forces, but there are again problems with representativeness.

Incubation time

Much work was done during the 1980's to elucidate the natural history of HIV infection, and especially the time from infection with HIV until the development of AIDS. One reason for this interest, apart from the obvious relevance to patients and physicians, is that the incubation time is an important variable if one wants to model the HIV epidemic. Since it can be assumed that most people with AIDS will be too ill to take part in the transmission of the virus, the incubation time would correspond to **D**, or the duration of infectivity, as discussed in Chapter 10. If one wants to calculate the basic reproductive rate for HIV infection using the formula:

$$R_o = \beta \times k \times D,$$

where β = risk of transmission per contact, **k** = number of contacts per time unit, and **D** = infectious period (measured in the same time unit as **k**), then one must know the value for **D**.

The first reports on incubation times were based on clinical cohorts, where seropositive patients were followed and the percentage who developed AIDS after one, two, three, etc. years of follow-up

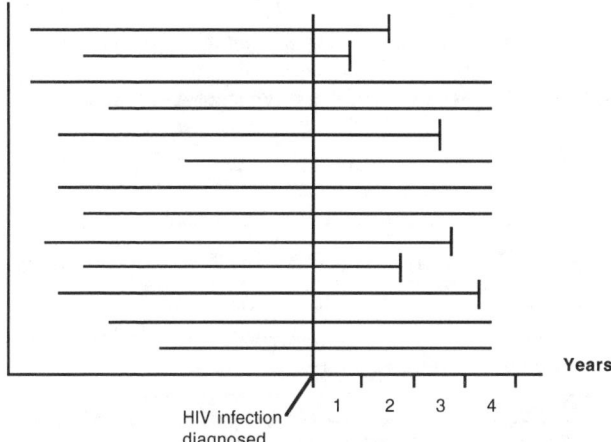

Fig. 19.1 *A schematic graph of a follow-up study of 13 HIV positive patients.*

were reported. This approach neglects that the patients had been infected for an unknown period of time before they were first seen in the clinic. Fig. 19.1 describes the situation:

Each line in the Figure represents a patient. The left end denotes actual date of infection (which is usually not known, neither to patient nor physician). For simplicity, we here assume that all these 13 patients with HIV infection were diagnosed at the same time, at the beginning of year one. The vertical bars at the right end of lines correspond to AIDS diagnosis in a patient.

A description of the rate of AIDS development in this cohort, would be that in the first year one out of 13 patients was diagnosed with AIDS, after two years a total of three patients, after three years a total of five, etc. These figures would not tell us anything about the real incubation time, since they fail to include the unknown time from infection to diagnosis of HIV positivity.

Other studies from the same time used a method that is also biased, but where this is not so easily detected.[1,2] They recognized the problem with unknown infection dates and looked only at AIDS cases who had been HIV-infected from a blood transfusion, and for whom the actual day of infection could be ascertained. The average time from transfusion to AIDS diagnosis could be calculated in this group of patients. However, this approach can only look at people who have developed AIDS when the study is made. At the same time there are also an unknown number of people infected via blood transfusion who have not developed AIDS, and in whom the HIV infection is not even diagnosed. The situation is shown in Fig. 19.2, where the left end of each line is again shows when a patient was infected, and where the vertical bars represent AIDS diagnoses:

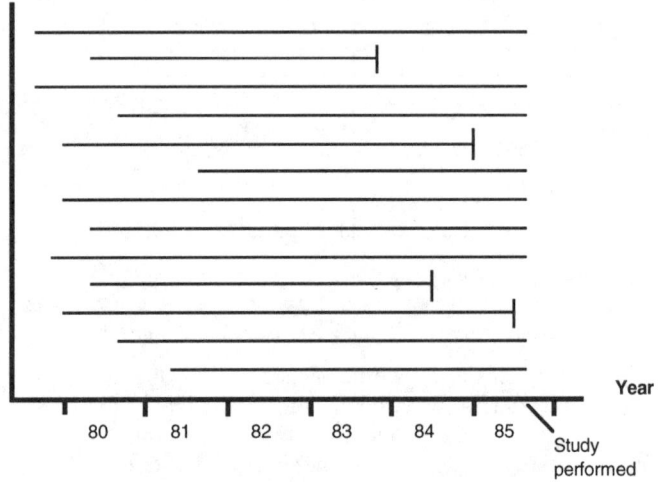

Fig. 19.2 *A schematic graph of a study reporting on incubation times for transfusion-associated AIDS cases.*

Here, we would know exactly when the four patients who had developed AIDS were infected. The average incubation time for them seems to be around four years. However, the other nine patients would be totally unknown to us, and we could not see that they still were asymptomatic HIV positive. The method described here will underestimate the true incubation time, since, in effect, it will pick up just those patients who have short incubation times.

The correct method to measure the incubation time is obviously to follow a cohort of seropositive people with known infection dates. This has been done for a group of homosexual men in San Francisco who had stored blood samples from a hepatitis B vaccine trial in the late 1970s, just when HIV started to spread there,[3] and also for haemophiliacs infected via factor concentrate, and for blood transfusion recipients in situations when all recipients from an infected donor could be traced and tested.[4] The present estimate of the median incubation time to AIDS is around 10 years, but there seems to be a wide range from short times of just one to two years up to 15 years or more in individual patients. The upper limit is still unknown, since the epidemic did not really start to spread to the parts of the world where studies like these can be performed with some ease until some 15 years ago. It may well be that a portion of the infected will never develop AIDS.

Factors influencing incubation time

Another issue has been if different patient groups have different incubation times. For example, early studies showed that blood transfusion recipients seemed to progress faster to AIDS than haemophiliacs. The curve in Fig. 19.3 shows the Kaplan–Meier plot for AIDS incidence in one group of transfusion recipients, and one group of haemophiliacs.[4]

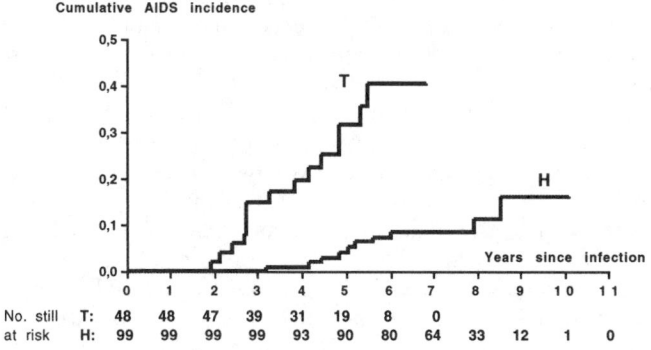

Fig. 19.3 *Kaplan–Meier plot of time from HIV infection to AIDS in one group of transfusion recipients (T) and one of haemophiliacs (H). Note the display of numbers still at risk along the time axis. (Figure based on two more years of follow-up than the data published in Giesecke* et al.[4])

However, this difference is possibly confounded by age, since transfusion recipients are on average much older than haemophiliacs. Recent studies indicate that age may be the main explanatory variable for length of incubation time, and that the period till half the infected have developed AIDS would be around 15 years in 20-year-olds, decreasing to seven to eight years in 65-year-olds.

Some other factors that have been discussed as risks for shorter incubation periods have been smoking, pregnancy, repeated other infections, and repeated exposure to HIV. There is, however, little hard data to substantiate these assumptions, and, again, such studies are made difficult by the fact that exact date of infection is known for so few patients.

Conversely, surveillance data now indicate that the time required for 50% of an infected group to develop AIDS is increasing, and it is generally believed that this is due to more and more HIV patients being treated with antivirals (mainly AZT) or with drugs that are prophylactic for opportunistic infections. Such treatment should postpone the onset of AIDS, which also means that the natural history of HIV infection can no longer be studied in countries with good access to health care.

'Surrogate' measures

The above discussion underlines the need for some proxy measure to determine approximately how long a patient has been infected. Also, the long course of an HIV infection makes clinical trials of antiviral drugs very cumbersome, since they will have to run for several years in order to register adequate number of 'events' (incident AIDS cases, deaths) in the trial groups, and some more immediate measure of disease progression would be very useful.

Several biological markers now exist that have been shown to be associated to disease progression in an HIV-infected patient. The one most widely used is the concentration of $CD4^+$ T-lymphocytes (T helper cells) in patient blood. These cells are infected by HIV, and their number decreases with time since infection. The normal value is around 800 cells/ml, and the risk of developing AIDS increases rapidly when the $CD4^+$ count goes below 200.

Even though the average downward progression in cohorts of HIV-positive subjects is quite well described, intersubject variations in base level still make it difficult to use the $CD4^+$ count for determining time since infection in a single individual. Instead, this proxy measure has found its greatest use in following the effect of treatment, where a patient's values are compared to his own pretreatment values.

The clinical use of $CD4^+$ counts has become so fundamental for treatment decisions that since 1993 the US AIDS case definition includes 'CD4-count below 200 in an HIV-positive person'.

Transmission routes

Not even the discoveries of the three major transmission routes for HIV infection: sexual intercourse, blood-to-blood contact, and mother-to-offspring could really be ascribed to formal epidemiological studies, but rather to growing collective evidence from clinical observations. More recently, however, proper attempts have been made to measure the risk of transmission through breast milk in cohort studies. Children born to known HIV-positive mothers have been followed, and the risk ratio of infection for breast-feeding versus bottle-feeding calculated.[5]

Such studies of breast-milk transmission have a potential problem with confounding: since HIV-positive mothers in developed countries are discouraged from breast-feeding their babies, the ones who still do may be different from other mothers in several respects, and this could play a role for transmission risks, even though it is unclear how.

Instead, the real role for epidemiology has been to show how HIV is *not* transmitted. It is obviously unethical to expose people to the virus in different ways to see if they acquire the infection or not, and we must make use of the information provided by the epidemic itself. Important issues in the early years were whether or not HIV could be transmitted in social contacts, such as hugging, kissing, or just sharing a glass. The possibility that mosquitoes could transfer the infection was also discussed.

In order to answer the first question, serological studies were made of family members to known HIV-positive patients. Those family members had often lived with the patient for a number of years before the infection was diagnosed, and had experienced the full range of social contacts with him/her. No transmissions to others than sexual partners were discovered in several hundred household contacts from different countries, which showed that the risk of social transmission must be very low.

Regarding the issue of mosquito-borne infection, early seroprevalence studies from Africa showed that prevalence was appreciable in infants, practically zero in ages five to adolescence, and then rising with increasing age into the 20's. If mosquitoes could transmit HIV, it would be highly unlikely that children were spared. The age pattern seems more consistent with transmission from mothers to the infants, and with a rise at the age of beginning sexual activity.

You might suggest that another good way of to discover possible routes of transmission would be to interview known HIV patients about how they might have become infected. This suggestion touches on a general problem with using surveillance data for infectious disease epidemiology: once a number of transmission routes for a disease have been scientifically established and known, the physician who diagnoses a case will ask the patient about these specific exposures, and be satisfied if the patient acknowledges any of them. For HIV surveillance this means that if the patient acknowledges intravenous drug use, then his infection will be ascribed to that transmission route. If he acknowledges sexual intercourse with another man his infection will be labelled 'homosexual transmission', and so on.

The problem with discovering new transmission routes for HIV through surveillance comes from the fact that almost all people who do not admit to any of the above specific risk behaviours will at least acknowledge heterosexual intercourse. Since this is a known risk factor, it will be assumed to be the actual route of transmission, and being such a common behaviour it could mask the existence of unknown routes. In a similar fashion, routine reporting may underestimate the extent of heterosexual transmission, since drug use and homosexual contact are commonly known to be stronger risk factors, which means that patients with these exposures will automatically be registered under those transmission categories.

Transmission risk

It has proven very difficult to assign exact numbers to the risk of HIV transmission in various situations, and especially to the risk in sexual contacts. It could admittedly be argued that exact values are of little practical importance: what difference would it make to the individual or to public health programmes whether the risk of transmission in vaginal intercourse was 0.1%, 1%, or even 10%? Would the exact level of risk really affect the health message? However, for the purpose of modelling the epidemic, these are important figures, corresponding to the variable β in the formula for the basic reproductive rate above.

Nonsexual transmission

Studies of recipients of blood transfusions from an infected donor have shown that the risk of infection is practically 100%. (In one instance when the risk seemed somewhat lower, it was found that one recipient never actually received the transfusion registered in the medical records.) These studies usually start with one diagnosed case of HIV infection in a recipient, then go on to find the donor, and finally trace all his/her other recipients, and could thus be regarded as retrospective cohort studies.

The risk of transmission in the health-care setting, mainly from accidental needle sticks, has been assessed in prospective cohort studies. Health-care workers who pricked themselves with a needle that had been used for a HIV-positive patient, or who cut themselves on contaminated glass or other sharp objects, were followed to see if they developed antibody to HIV. Obviously, the estimated risk would be too high if people who were already infected with HIV when the accident occurred were included in the cohorts, and most studies have stipulated that a so-called base line blood sample must be taken directly after the accident.

The probability that an HIV-positive pregnant woman will transmit the infection to her child, either during pregnancy or at birth, can also be assessed in prospective cohort studies, where babies to known positive mothers are followed after birth.[6] This seems straightforward enough, and I should refrain from going into the real subtleties of HIV epidemiology in this chapter, but I will point out just one in this context: who are the mothers whose HIV status is known prior to delivery? Is there anything special about them that could bias the selection of known positive women? Well, one common reason for being tested is that the woman has previously born a child who developed AIDS. If it were that some women are at greater risk to transmit HIV, then they would have a higher probability of already being diagnosed. Those women would thus be over-represented in the original cohort, and the sample would not be representative of all HIV-positive pregnant women. Such a selection bias should render the calculated overall transmission risk too high. This example shows that one cannot be too careful when one looks for bias (or confounding). Alternatively, it might be seen as a demonstration that there is a limit to how far one should pursue one's methodological rigour, especially since the last decimal of the calculated risk probably has very little practical relevance anyway.

Sexual transmission

The main problem when studying sexual transmission is the long incubation time. For most HIV patients it is unknown when or by whom they were infected. Our knowledge of transmission probability comes mainly from the study of couples, where one partner is discovered to be positive. When this partner's date of infection is known, as in transfusion recipients or many haemophiliac men, it becomes possible to calculate the risk per 'couple year' by testing the other partner and combining a number of such couples in a retrospective cohort study. It must of course be assumed that the other partner could not have become infected by someone else.

If the couples are asked about their average frequency of intercourse, it becomes possible to estimate a risk per intercourse. This, however, assumes that the risk is equal in each intercourse, and also that this risk is similar for all couples. The virus could be transmitted very soon in some couples, whereas in others it may not be transmitted at all. Some studies indicate that some persons transmit HIV very easily, but little is known about whether some people are especially susceptible.

Prospective studies of risk of sexual transmission are difficult, since most couples where one partner is positive and one negative will change to safer sexual behaviour, by using condoms more consistently than before. This means that the assessed risk will no longer correspond to the more 'natural' situation, where the two partners' HIV status is unknown to them.

Several couple studies have showed that the risk of transmission increases if the infective partner has developed symptoms of HIV infection. Such studies have a major problem with confounding, however: if the infective partner is symptomatic, he/she has probably been infected for a long time, and the couple has probably had sexual intercourse many times. An asymptomatic infective person may have become infected recently, and will not have exposed his/her partner so many times.

One approach to measuring infectivity in sexual intercourse is to use partner notification data. If patients diagnosed with HIV infection are asked about their partners, and these partners can be located and agree to being tested for HIV, it becomes possible to calculate risks of transmission in different types of partnerships. The necessary prerequisite is that the infectious status of both partners at the time they started their relationship can be assessed retrospectively.

In one such study in Sweden,[7] 365 newly diagnosed HIV patients were interviewed about sexual partners. These interviews resulted in description of 246 hetero- or homosexual partnerships with partners of known HIV status, and for 100 of these it could be established that one partner had been positive and one negative when they first met. This was mostly done from results of previous HIV tests, but also from the contact tracing itself: if a positive index patient had only had one positive partner and all other partners where tested negative, then this must be the source of the infection.

These 100 partnerships, in which the partners were originally *discordant* regarding HIV status made up a cohort in which risk of infection could be studied. HIV was transmitted in 30 partnerships, for an overall attack rate of 30%. Since anal intercourse had been suggested to carry a higher attack rate than vaginal, and since other studies had shown increased risk of transmission from patients with symptomatic infection, these two factors were analysed together in two combined 2 × 2 tables (Table 19.1).

Table 19.1 Risk of sexual HIV transmission by type of intercourse and by stage of disease in the infective partner. Figures in parentheses are 95% confidence intervals. Source: Giesecke et al.[7]

Stage, infective partner	Type of intercourse	Partners infected	Partners not infected	Transmission probability, %
No symptom	Heterosexual (vaginal)	11	43	20 (9–31)
	Homosexual (anal)	10	18	36 (18–54)
Any symptom	Heterosexual	2	5	29 (0–62)
	Homosexual	7	4	64 (36–92)

This way of combining two tables in one is an example of a simple stratification for a confounder, which in this case would be stage of infection. You can see that 11/28 (39%) of the initially infected homosexual men had symptoms, versus only 7/54 (13%) of the heterosexual subjects. If this fact had not been controlled for, the difference in transmission risk between the two types of intercourse would have seemed even greater.

There has been much debate about the role of other STDs in HIV transmission. Does a person who has another STD transmit HIV more readily, and will a HIV-negative person with an STD become infected more easily? This is also an issue where confounding is a problem: many case-control studies have shown that HIV-positive patients have higher prevalence of other STDs, or higher seroprevalence of markers for past such infections, than HIV-negative controls. The problem is that all STDs are acquired in the same fashion, and that people whose sexual behaviour put them at high risk for acquiring gonorrhoea, syphilis, herpes, etc., will be just the same people who are at risk for becoming infected with HIV. The confounding comes from the fact that when one divides people into those who have or do not have different STDs, one will put the people with high-risk sexual behaviour in the 'have' group, just as discussed in Chapter 4. The best study of an STD as cofactor for HIV transmission is the one from Nairobi used as an example in Chapter 5.

Mixing patterns

Mixing patterns obviously play a major role for the shape of the AIDS epidemic. They also become important for estimates of the magnitude of different risk factors. Several case-control studies correlate the risk of HIV infection to the number of sexual partners that the person has had. Others calculate the odds for infection according to type of sexual contact, for example, oral versus anal intercourse. Most of these studies implicitly assume that exposure is constant over time and uniformly distributed across all partners.

Studies of the first type may ascribe an increase in prevalence to a corresponding increase in average number of partners. However, if prevalence rises in the studied group, that means that they will also infect their partners to greater degree, which in turn leads to a higher risk per contact for the study subjects. This interaction between the studied group and their partners is actually quite complex, especially if one wants to analyse the pattern over time. If you remember the example about herpes simplex type 2 infection in pregnant women in Chapter 8, we said that increasing seroprevalence at a certain age over a 20-year period could be due to a higher number of partners before becoming pregnant. However, it is just as possible that the proportion of all men who were infectious had increased with time, so that the risk per partner had also increased. In fact, since we did observe an increased seroprevalence in the women, this must also have led to an increased prevalence in the men who were their partners. Without corresponding seroprevalence data for men, it becomes impossible to determine which of the two explanations for the increase in women should be more correct.

The risk of infection associated with different behaviours of course also depends on the prevalence of infection in the presumptive partners. Assume that a certain kind of sexual behaviour is very common in one group, where HIV prevalence just happens to be high (e.g. because the virus was introduced very early), and that another kind of behaviour is common in another group with low seroprevalence. The behaviour in the first group will now appear to carry a much higher transmission risk than the other, just because the susceptible members of that group will have a higher probability of meeting an infected partner.[8]

Both these examples are somewhat theoretical, but they point to problems that can be overlooked by epidemiologists who are not used to thinking in terms of infectivity and mixing patterns.

For the modellers, the above discussions imply that we can get useful values for β and $\mathbf{D}$, even if we have to use a whole array of different β's for different types of contact. Also, we might have to assume that β increases, for example, when a person is infected with an STD. However, the remaining problem is $\mathbf{k}$, number of contacts per time unit. If the population were neatly divided into distinct compartments, such as injecting drug users, homosexual men, heterosexual men and women, etc., we could possibly arrive at some value of $\mathbf{k}$ for each of them. The problem is that the compartments are not distinct, and we know very little about how often contacts occur between them. The very simple model of Chapter 10 does not account for this situation, and it remains a problem even for much more elaborate and complex models.

The figures given in this chapter may, however, be used for a simple example of the use of the formula for R_0. The table on sexual transmission above gives the risk in a heterosexual relationship with an asymptomatic HIV positive person to be about 20% $(=\beta)$. The average time from infection till the development of AIDS seems to be around 10 years $(=\mathbf{D})$. What rate of partner change per year $(=\mathbf{k})$ would be needed in a heterosexual population in order to maintain HIV endemic? The formula would become:

$$R_0 = 0.2 \times \mathbf{k} \times 10 = 2 \times \mathbf{k}$$

In an endemic situation, $R_0 = 1$, which would give a value for $\mathbf{k}$ of 0.5. This is equal to stating that if people changed partners on the average every second year, then HIV would remain endemic in this population. If rate of partner change was higher, then there would be an epidemic situation.

Is it infectious?

The debate about the aetiology of AIDS has continued since the disease was first named, and some scientists maintain that AIDS is not caused by HIV infection, but rather by a particular lifestyle, by repeated other infections, and possibly by poppers. One Canadian study attempted to refute these hypotheses.[9]

From 1982 to 1984, 715 homosexual men were recruited into a cohort from six general practices in Vancouver. They were followed up twice yearly until 1986 and yearly thereafter for a median follow-up time of 8.6 years. At each visit they completed a questionnaire on lifestyle and illnesses. Initially, 237 of the men were HIV positive, and another 128 seroconverted during the study.

AIDS cases were diagnosed in the six participating clinics, but since some cohort members could have been diagnosed elsewhere, the British Columbia provincial and the Canadian national AIDS registries were also searched for AIDS cases among the participants.

By April, 1992, 136 cases of AIDS had been diagnosed in the cohort, all of them in the group that either was positive initially or had seroconverted. One hundred and three of the cohort members had died, 101 in the seropositive and two in the seronegative group. Ninety-five of the deaths were AIDS-related, all of these were in the seropositive group. There thus seemed to be a very strong relationship between 'being HIV positive' and developing AIDS. Theoretically, however, if seropositivity was strongly associated with some other, behavioural risk factor, this could be an effect of confounding, although confounders with this magnitude of association are very rare indeed.

In order to compare distribution of behavioural risk factors the cohort was divided into three groups (see Table 19.2): seropositive men who developed AIDS, seropositive men who had not developed AIDS, and seronegative men. The percentages of men in each group who reported ever having used poppers, ever having used illicit drugs, and having had anal intercourse in more than 25% of all sexual encounters are given in the Table.

Table 19.2 Percentages of homosexual men in three groups reporting three different types of risk-related behaviour. The first group of men were HIV positive and had been diagnosed with AIDS, the second were HIV positive only, and the third were HIV negative. Source: Schechter et al.[9]

Behaviour	HIV+/AIDS+ (n=136)	HIV+/AIDS− (n=229)	HIV− (n=350)
Poppers	88	88	56
Illicit drugs	75	80	74
Anal sex	72	82	58

There was thus no difference between the two groups of seropositive men, and the fact that some of them had progressed to AIDS and some not could hardly be explained by any of these risk behaviours. That the seronegative group reported lower prevalence of these behaviours is hardly surprising, since risk of being HIV positive has been shown to be related to all these three behaviours. However, these behaviours seem common enough in the third group to make it very unlikely that not one single case of AIDS should have appeared in that group if these factors had been involved in the causation of AIDS.

Summary

The study of the epidemiology of HIV infection gives a good list of examples of the problems attached to epidemiology in general. The long, asymptomatic incubation period makes surveillance difficult. Strategies to assess prevalence are influenced by selection biases.

The incubation time distribution can be studied in cohorts, but it is difficult to assemble unbiased cohorts of patients with known infection dates.

Concerning transmission routes, the main achievement of epidemiology has been to clarify how HIV is *not* transmitted. However, since almost all of the presently known seropositive patients have been exposed to at least one acknowledged transmission route, routine surveillance now has little power to detect additional routes, if such exist.

The actual risk of transmission is also best assessed in different types of cohort studies. Studies of cofactors for transmission, such as stage of infection or concurrent STDs, have some problems with confounding.

Mixing patterns influence calculations of risks and odds in ways that seldom are a problem for the epidemiology of noninfectious diseases.

References

1. Lui K-J, Lawrence DN, Morgan WM, Peterman TA, Haverkos HW, Bregman DJ. A model-based approach for estimating the mean incubation period of transfusion-associated acquired immunodeficiency syndrome. *Proc Natl Acad Sci USA* 1986; **83**: 3051–55.

2. Medley GF, Anderson RM, Cox DR, and Billard L. Incubation period of AIDS in patients infected via blood transfusion. *Nature* 1987; **328**: 719–21.

3. Bacchetti P, Moss AR. Incubation period of AIDS in San Francisco. *Nature* 1989; **338**: 251–53.

4. Giesecke J, Scalia-Tomba G-P, Berglund O, Berntorp E, Schulman S, Stigendal L. Incidence of symptoms and AIDS in 146 Swedish haemophiliacs and blood transfusion recipients infected with human immunodeficiency virus. *Br Med J* 1988; **297**: 99–102.

5. Dunn DT, Newell ML, Ades AE, Peckham CS. Risk of HIV-1 transmission through breast-feeding. *Lancet* 1992: **340**; 585–88.

6. European Collaborative Study. Risk factors for mother-to-child transmission of HIV-1. *Lancet* 1992: **339**; 1007–12.

7. Giesecke J, Ramstedt K, Granath F, Ripa T, Rådö G, Westrell M. Partner notification as a method for research into HIV epidemiology – behaviour changes, transmission risks, and incidence measures. *AIDS* 1992; **6**: 101–107.

8. Jacquez JA, Simon CP, Koopman J, Sattenspiel L, Percy T. Modeling and analyzing HIV transmission: The effect of contact patterns. *Math Biosci* 1988; **92**: 119–99.

9. Schechter MT, Craib KJP, Gelmon KA, Montaner JSG, Le TN, O'Shaughnessy MV. HIV-1 and the aetiology of AIDS. *Lancet* 1993; **341**: 658–59.

Index